CONTENTS

INTRODUCTION

My name is Gavin and I am a personal trainer. I created the Twelve Week Fitness and Nutrition Programme, tailoring one for women and one for men – both with amazing results.

The Twelve Week Fitness and Nutrition Programme for Men has been designed to show you how to change your body and lifestyle for the better in just 12 weeks. This book is for those who want to change, and change is inevitable. How much you change is up to you.

HOW DOES THE CHALLENGE WORK?

I noticed that most other 12-week programmes available on the market showed very unrealistic 'before' and 'after' shots, completely unachievable for the average person. I wanted to design a simple, achievable programme that anyone could follow in their own home, and that would be believable and achievable for anyone willing to give it a try. It was important not to have any of the photos retouched, so what you see in this book is 100 per cent real. No gimmicks, no airbrushing, real results.

I used my home gym and bike, home health checks (glucose test, cholesterol test and blood pressure kit), other health tests readily available on the Internet (fat percentage monitor, callipers, tape measure and peak flow meter), bleep tests, home-made postural examination with a plumb line and home-made photo studio.

There are over 60 different workouts in this book, with pictures of the training, exercises, running,

and cycling showing my progression throughout the 12-week programme. Over 80 of the exercises performed in this book are illustrated, each with a label explaining its purpose and how to perform it effectively.

WILL THE 12-WEEK PROGRAMME WORK FOR ME?

Believe it or not, it would work for anybody who wants to give it a go.

I have trained clients from all walks of life for years, ranging from Hollywood stars to triathletes. The Twelve Week Fitness and Nutrition Programme for Men contains the knowledge that I have passed on to them, and now I can pass it on to you in the same way.

HOW DID I DO THIS?

I needed to start my training slowly and build it up gradually as I hadn't trained for such a long time throughout my fattening-up process. This will be

No gimmicks
No airbrushing

GAVIN MOREY

B L O O M S B U R Y

LONDON · NEW DELHI · NEW YORK · SYDNEY

Published by Bloomsbury Publishing Plc
50 Bedford Square
London WC1B 3DP
www.bloomsbury.com

Bloomsbury is a trademark of Bloomsbury Publishing Plc

First edition 2014

Copyright © 2014 Gavin Morey

ISBN (paperback): 978-1-4081-9636-6
ISBN (ePdf): 978-1-4081-9638-0
ISBN (EPUB): 978-1-4081-9637-3

A CIP catalogue record for this book is available from the British Library.

Acknowledgements
Cover photograph © Shutterstock
Inside photographs © the author, except pages 68, 128, 180 and 214 © Grant Pritchard; and food photographs in chapter 6 © Shutterstock
Illustrations by David Gardner
Commissioned by Kirsty Schaper

This book is produced using paper that is made from wood grown in managed, sustainable forests. It is natural, renewable and recyclable. The logging and manufacturing processes conform to the environmental regulations of the country of origin.

Typeset in URW Grotesk Light by seagulls.net
Printed and bound in China by C&C Offset Printing Co

10 9 8 7 6 5 4 3 2 1

the case for most people who lead a fairly inactive lifestyle. I started off working on my upper body and running to introduce my body to training again. I then chose to weight train to give my body some shape, size and mass. The cardio training improved my fitness level, enabled me to lose body fat and get healthy again. And finally I chose circuits to lose further body fat, help with my cardio and increase muscular endurance.

This training was a major factor in getting my body back into shape, but without following a sensible nutrition plan the results would not be so impressive. The nutrition plan is just as important as the training, if not more so.

INJURY AND DISCLAIMER

Muscles and injuries are my field of expertise, but before you begin any hard and strenuous exercise you should consult a GP. This is only to have reassurance from the medical field. When I started my 12-week programme I saw my GP to explain to him what I had planned, and also because I wanted to find out if the home testing kits were accurate enough to base my health and fitness results on.

ACKNOWLEDGEMENTS

I don't know where to start, but I would like to thank my family and friends for all their support throughout the past five years on the making of these books. It has been a long and hard process, but it has been well worth it in the end.

I have had a lot of help from my mum and dad; you both mean the world to me. To my brothers, Chris, Rob and Aaron, I would like to thank you for keeping me grounded and helping me with the books and website. Thanks to my friend Simon for being there for the past 12 years with all of my silly ideas and enterprises, and to Gav for training with me and keeping me on track all the way to the end. I would also just like to say thank you to Fred for training with me throughout the 12 weeks and helping me with all of my business concerns.

Finally, to my beautiful and devoted wife, Alison, You have given me so much help and support throughout the years in getting these books to this stage, I am forever in your debt. However, not only have you brought the books to life but you have given us the biggest gift anyone could ever ask for, our gorgeous little boy Morgen. I love you both so much, and words can never express what I truly feel. Thank you, and I love you so much.

HEALTHY LIFESTYLE VERSUS UNHEALTHY LIFESTYLE

01

This book is here to show you the truth behind poor fitness programmes, faddy diets, fake photos and imagined results. To achieve your ultimate goal it takes effort, hard training, a healthy balanced diet, lifestyle changes and commitment.

In this chapter we cover at how many times you will be training a week, look behind the scenes of my own training progress, as well as seeing why I decided to put on two stone for the sake of the Twelve Week Fitness and Nutrition Programme in the first place.

I wanted to show clearly the progress of my training through photos and weekly fitness and health tests. Also, I needed to know that I could complete the plan myself first. I thought if you could see how I completed the plan and exactly what I went through, it would be more achievable for you. It's the case of practising what I preach to my clients and doing it myself in exactly the same way.

BEFORE THE CHALLENGE
FIVE MONTHS OF FATTENING-UP

Surprisingly, for the first month or so it was heaven. It was as if I was on holiday, but it wasn't long before I started feeling the negative effects.

The worst moment with regard to my fitness came when I took one of my clients for a physical training (PT) session and asked him to do as many push-ups as possible in a minute after training for over 45 minutes. I was asked to join in and was surprised when my client beat me quite easily. (He had not trained for over 20 years due to a back injury.) He beat me after only a year of training, and when I was only three months into my fattening-up process.

HOW DID I FEEL PUTTING THE WEIGHT ON?

It wasn't long before I started feeling tired, bored of not doing anything, weak and pathetic. I also felt extremely self-conscious, fat, lazy and useless. My confidence plummeted.

My changing posture started causing me lower back pain from an earlier scuba diving accident. I had started getting hyperlordosis. My core muscles were becoming very weak, which was resulting in my back pain.

My skin was in a terrible state too, with spots all over my face and body. And I had gained two stone in body fat. I couldn't fit into my clothes comfortably and hated getting changed in front of people.

WHAT DID I EAT DIFFERENTLY WHILE GETTING FAT?

To fatten up I drank a lot of sweet fizzy drinks. For breakfast I would have sugary cereal with semi-skimmed milk and for lunch I would have two rounds of sandwiches or rolls with pre-made fillings. I would then eat pasta and pizzas for dinner followed by dessert, which mainly consisted of cake and ice cream.

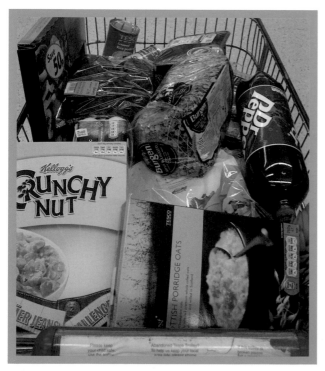

How to put weight on healthily?

I snacked on crisps and chocolate or muesli bars, which are full of sugar and not very healthy. With regard to alcohol, I was not a big drinker before my plan so I didn't change this in any way – I wanted to gain two stone in a fairly healthy way to avoid ruining my internal organs.

BEHIND THE SCENES

This is as real as it gets, taking you into my life, with real pictures and results to show you that you can do anything you want if you put your mind to it.

I found it hard looking through various health and fitness books that show amazing results in just two weeks. These books promise you the earth, and to follow their diet normally consists of you following a bodybuilder's pre-contest diet. Of course this type of diet works, but trust me, I have trained a fair few amateur bodybuilders in my time, and they do not follow this type of plan all year round.

When I looked through the 'before' and 'after' pictures of these people in health and fitness books, I noticed that the photos did not look realistic. They either looked like they were completely different people, heavily airbrushed, or that the photos have been taken after a far greater length of time than was being claimed. Also, some of the before photos were of extremely poor quality, and in the 'after' photo it clearly showed that they had had a make-over to look flawless under great studio lighting.

On a serious note, it is never good to lose weight too quickly as your body needs time to adapt to its new routine. Remember, with the yo-yo diet you will always end up putting more body fat on than when you started trying to lose it.

This book is for all those people who want to see a real change with real results, true-life photographs with no airbrushing, and simple no-gimmick training that I have road-tested – if I can do it, so can you.

FAKE TAN OR REAL TAN?

I have never used fake tan in my life, and I'm not going to start now. If you notice me getting a tan during my 12-week plan, this is because I was both training and writing this book outside as much as I could throughout the summer months.

REAL PICTURES OR AIRBRUSHED PICTURES?

Airbrushing is one thing that I'm dead against. I need you, as the reader, to understand what it actually takes to get into shape, and if I ended up using airbrushing I would be cheating myself and cheating you by showing something that cannot be sensibly achieved.

The style of these pictures is based on the photos you normally see in fitness magazines. The difference with mine is that when you look closely you will see some of my flaws and blemishes – no airbrushing.

Week 1   Week 12

HAIR TODAY GONE TOMORROW

I shaved some of my body hair every week to show clearly exactly what happens to your body when you follow the 12-week programme, so that you can clearly see the change in muscularity. If I had decided to keep all my body hair, you wouldn't be able to see what happened to my body and how my muscles developed in terms of density, size, shape and separation, while also losing weight.

Please note, you do not have to shave your body to get the same results that I did. Just enjoy the training.

Hairy

Shaved

Hairy

Shaved

These photos were taken around week 12 in preparation for my *GQ* magazine photo shoot.

PHOTOGRAPHS

I chose to take photographs weekly to show you exactly what happened to my body and what could happen to yours. Also, I wanted the weekly photos to prove that the before and after photos were not separated by a longer period, so that you can follow my process with accuracy.

I took the photos at the same time of the morning. This ensured my body was not pumped in any way and gave the truest results possible.

I decided not to use a professional photographer, but to take the photographs myself with the help of friends. This provides you with real non-professional photographs that do not make me look as though I am wearing make-up.

PUMPED OR NOT?

My brother asked me once, 'Are you pumping up before the end photos to get the best results?', to which I replied, 'No'. So he said, 'Prove it' – and I think I have.

If I pumped myself up on every test day, all of my tests would be greatly out and noticeably so. My results and measurements would have been more impressive and I would probably have an extra inch on the measurements for my arms, chest, legs, etc. So to keep it real for you, my pictures and measurements are of me standing cold and relaxed.

I took the photos on week 12 as normal, cold and relaxed, and then I went into the gym and pumped myself up. You can notice a massive difference after I'd worked out – not only are my muscles all pumped and looking a lot bigger and with more separation, but I also look more impressive all over. All the pictures you see throughout the book are of me relaxed and not pumped up.

SUPPLEMENTS

I'm not sure why so many books say you have to take shakes and/or supplements to reach your dream physique. That is a load of rubbish, and it angers me because this is not the case. Taking supplement/ shakes will make reaching your goal slightly easier

Not pumped

Pumped

You can see from the pumped picture after I finished around 100 pull-ups and lifting some weights, the greater definition and muscle mass in my back.

because you won't need to cook or eat as much, but it is definitely not healthier for you.

If you do choose to take supplements alongside your fitness and nutrition plan, please buy the best quality ones you can. I'm not against supplements, just the misuse of them. If you use them sensibly, they can aid in achieving your dream physique, but only if used alongside a balanced and healthy diet. Provided they are accredited, you should achieve excellent results.

In the next chapter you will get to know your body inside and out, by recognising your body's health signs. You will start to understand how a poor diet or deficiency in vitamins or minerals can affect you. If you are suffering from a deficiency, then by all means either try eating the right foods or take supplements. However, following the 12-week programme should prove to you that you don't have to use supplements and protein/meal replacement shakes to get to where you want to be. It just takes the right training, nutrition, commitment, motivation and determination, all of which have to be fun.

FOLLOWING THE BOOK

Use this book and the training diaries as guidance and reference, to show how hard you should train throughout the 12 weeks. You will be able to note

Not pumped

Pumped

To be honest I never thought there would be such a dramatic change standing relaxed while pumped, but when you see it next to the photo of me when I have just got up, you can see a complete change in my muscles.

down in your own training diary, which is provided, what you have been doing, the times you have been training, the weights you have been lifting, the training RPE (rating perceived exertion), etc. When following the workouts, each exercise is in order so please follow it step by step to know what to do first. The training diary is your very own fitness programme, which you can take everywhere. I even took mine on holiday. I used my training diary as a progress report showing me what I was running or lifting, so the next time I attempted to do the same exercise I would want to try and improve on it no matter how small the difference.

At the start of every week's training overview, you can jot down your feelings in your own personal diary. You will also notice the tests you need to take to monitor your progress every week, and again you can compare your results next to mine. There are monthly tests for your glucose and cholesterol levels, postural analysis, etc., as well as the weekly tests of measurement, weight, body mass index (BMI), etc.

TRAINING

You will begin your training by exercising just three times for the first week. As the weeks go by, the number of training days will increase. I have done it this way to prevent overtraining, as well as giving you lots of rest days to allow your body to recover.

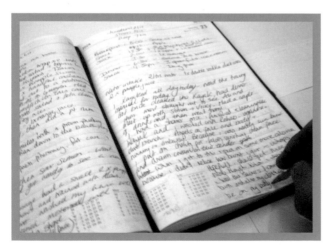

I wrote in my health diary how I was feeling about my eating, as well as other personal accounts, to help me write these books.

Near the middle, and towards the end of the programme, I have used shock tactics in the weight training sessions to try and get the most out of your muscles. You will also notice the mileage on the running and cycling picks up throughout the 12-week programme. This should enable you to run a 10-miler at the end quite easily, as well as cycling over 20 miles.

Important note: I didn't train legs with weights at the beginning of the programme on purpose, due to the amount of exercise you will do through running and circuit training. Once your legs have built up some strength and endurance, we then move on to developing size, mass and strength.

You will also notice there isn't a training session specifically for arms until you're a third of the way through the programme. This is due to the amount of stress that will be placed upon them at the beginning of your training session, with your chest, back and shoulder sessions. Your arms will be getting bigger and stronger from this alone. Later you will weight train your arms, and this will be just as hard as training any other muscle group.

HOW MANY TIMES WILL YOU EXERCISE?

In total I exercised 63 out of 84 days. I exercised on average five times a week, but it would vary as the weeks went by. For instance, the first week it was only three times, and by the end of the 12 weeks it was seven times a week.

On average, your training per week will be:

- 2 × cardio
- 2 × weight training
- 1 × circuit training

HOW MANY REST DAYS?

On average you will have two days off per week. I had 21 rest days over the 12 weeks.

HOW LONG ARE THE WORKOUT SESSIONS?

At the end, the average time for the workout was 1 hour 20 minutes. Of course, this is an average. I had short training sessions of 20 minutes and long sessions of up to five hours (walking/kayaking). I usually worked out at 6.00 p.m. in the evening, and when I worked out in the morning it would normally be at 8.15 a.m., but you can do the workouts at any time.

HOLIDAY AND TRAINING

It is still possible to be good, eat well and train hard when you're away on holiday. I had a long-weekend break, during which I did lots of walking and even found a gym at which to train in the morning. Look at Chapter 3 on healthy eating to see how to choose the right meals when you eat out.

For the training I did the best I could with the facilities I had, such as using a chair for dips and the staircase for hill sprints. The most important thing was that I always walked everywhere. I would walk up and down the stairs instead of taking lifts – I even walked up the escalators. I also had a 30-minute walk to and from work, and all of this helped regulate my weight loss.

CHEAT DAYS, TRAINING AND NUTRITION

The purpose of the nutritional programme is not about dieting or dictating what you can and cannot eat. Its aim is not to reduce the amounts of food you eat, or even to deprive you of vital carbohydrates or fat, but to show that you can achieve a good physique by following a healthy plan that contains all your nutritional requirements.

With regard to the fitness side, I listened to whether my body was giving me signs indicating that I was too stressed or overdoing things, and I would then change what I was doing. This is why you have so many rest days at the beginning, to prepare your body for the increase in training over the 12 weeks.

TRAINING THROUGH ALL CONDITIONS

You may come up with all sorts of excuses why you can't train, but when you really want something badly enough, nothing should stand in your way.

SETTING GOALS

I always tell my clients about the importance of setting goals. This will motivate you all the way to the end, and push you to limits you might never have thought possible. When choosing your goals you should aim big, such as being able to run 10 miles. You should then have lots of little goals in between to keep you motivated and on track.

My big goal was to get the best results possible in the 12 weeks, and my little goals were all the training days during those 12 weeks. In reading this book it means that you have chosen your big goal. Use everything from this book to guide you towards achieving it.

HOW DID YOU GET THROUGH THE TRAINING ON BAD DAYS?

I trained through the rough days by thinking of the end result. I also tried to train with friends as much as possible so we could motivate each other. My best friend and I have a couple of sayings from when we were teenagers: 'harder, faster, quicker, more', and 'bigger, better, best'. When we say these words we are normally taking the mick out of each other, but the words do represent training and what we are trying to achieve.

DOMS – DELAYED ONSET MUSCLE SORENESS

Often felt 24 to 72 hours after exercising, DOMS can cause pain, discomfort, stiffness and strength loss, which generally subsides within two to three days. Although the precise cause is still unknown, a theory recently developed states that DOMS is caused by the breakdown of muscular fibres. This is particularly apparent in strength/resistance programmes. The breakdown occurs due to stress and allows the muscles to grow stronger and larger.

Try not to worry if you have DOMS. When you read through my diary you will see I suffered from DOMS on a regular basis.

REMEMBER THESE SIMPLE STEPS TO HELP COMBAT DOMS:

1. Stretch in between sets while exercising.
2. Stretch at the end of the programme.
3. Stretch the muscles suffering from DOMS at least 6–12 times a day.
4. If you're really sore do not exercise your muscles, take a day off to allow them to recover.

OVERTRAINING

We start nice and slowly with the training to prevent overtraining. You don't want to exhaust your body so you can't complete the 12-week programme. That is why the first three weeks are nice and easy, with the workouts gradually increasing in intensity over the 12 weeks.

Overtraining comes from training beyond the body's ability to recover. It can come from training too hard or too long without the adequate recovery and rest. If left too long this will backfire – it will decrease your performance in training and you will start to lose your physique.

The signs of overtraining:

- Feeling tired and drained.
- Lack of energy and the feeling of not wanting to train.
- Pain in your muscles and possibly joints.
- Drop in performance – diminished power, speed, strength and endurance.
- Lack of concentration.

TREATING OVERTRAINING

The only way to counteract overtraining is to stop all training and exercise and rest for at least three days, or until you feel that your body and mind are functioning properly together. When you rest, remember that it should be complete rest, and you should drink plenty of water and eat a little more food than normal. This will help your muscles recover back to their full capacity again, and then you are ready to resume training. When you do go back into training, make sure that you take it easy for the first week and then gradually increase your performance.

Just look at the state of me after a 6-mile run in the rain.

KNOWING YOUR BODY INSIDE AND OUT

02

It is important to know your body inside and out. What is normal for you may not be normal for someone else, and vice versa. Everyone can say that they have noticed things about their body that were not normal for them at one time or another. Your body talks to you all the time, perhaps only in subtle measures, but by learning to read these signals it will enable you to act on anything that may be upsetting your well-being or disturbing your equilibrium.

The signs may be small, and you may feel that they are even unimportant, like having yellow fingers, for example. This could simply be a result of nicotine discolouration – however, it could also be a warning sign for a disorder in your liver or lungs. Try not to take anything for granted.

Knowing how to differentiate between these small signals before they turn into the actual symptoms of a disorder is a delicate matter, and should not be rushed. The following information is an easy reference guide to highlight some things that may be troubling you, and how you can watch out for signs of poor health in your own body.

TONGUE

We can detect a lot about the health of a person by looking at aspects of their tongue, such as changes to the shape, size, colour, texture and coating. In fact, the tongue is still used today in Chinese medicine to help diagnose various health concerns. The tongue is covered with several types of papillae or nodules that continually shed and grow like hair, making it a great source of information about our health.

This is a guide for a healthy tongue:

- Size and shape – normal and proportionate to the body
- Colour – salmon or pinky red shade
- Texture – smooth with no marks or cracks
- Coating – thin, white, moist coating across the whole tongue

Here are some things to look out for when investigating your tongue. These could be caused by different conditions or could well be an indication of possible problems within certain body systems. Remember, this is just a guideline.

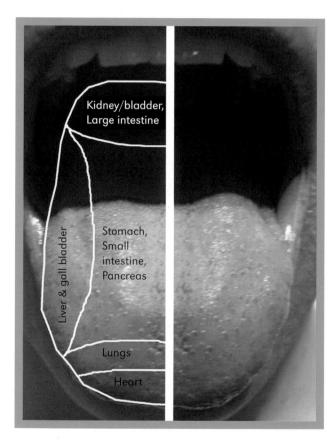

Week 1 – please note the teeth marks on the side of my tongue and the slightly red tip. Both of these signs indicate poor nutrition, something that the 12-week nutrition programme helped me to alleviate by eating a healthy balanced diet.

SIZE AND SHAPE

Big and unusually red – the protective papillae could be being damaged, for example, by teeth or dentures rubbing on the tongue.

Swollen – this could be due to poor digestion. For swollen sides of the tongue, it could be that the liver is being overworked, or there is a problem within the gallbladder.

COLOUR

Unusually red – possibly acute fever. If it is also smooth, it may indicate a vitamin B12 deficiency or an intestinal disorder where nutrients are not being adequately absorbed.

Red tip – indication of depression, a lack of sleep or stress.

Pale – possible lack of nutrients within the body such as vitamin B12 or folic acid. It may also be caused by a hormone imbalance.

Purple – poor circulation, poor nutrition or a lack of vitamin B complex and minerals.

TEXTURE

Peeling – dry mouth or a deficiency in vitamin B.

Teeth marks – normally occurs with a swollen tongue and could suggest digestion problems.

Scrotal tongue – an indication of an infection or poor nutrition.

Groovy tongue – something people are usually born with, and may not be noticed right away. It tends to become more noticeable as you age.

COATING

White – indication of the recovery from a recent fever or a poor diet lacking in fibre.

Black – possible reaction to antibiotics or to stomach medication. Poor oral hygiene, smoking, excessive use of mouthwash, infection, digestion or poorly managed diabetes may also cause this.

Brown and yellow – trapped bacteria and food or excessive smoking and coffee. Yellow coating is normally seen with a red tip.

TEETH AND GUMS

We all want those pearly white teeth and healthy gums to give the biggest and best smile imaginable. As a rule, I will usually brush my teeth twice a day, but please note that if you are following the information below visit your dentist when it is next convenient.

Here are some things to look out for when investigating your teeth and gums. These could be caused by different conditions, or could well be an indication of possible future dental problems, so please consult your dentist if you have any concerns at all.

TEETH

Sensitive – caused by the thinning of your enamel layer (the outer layer that protects your inner dentine), which causes the dentine underneath to become exposed. Dental erosion, gum recession, gum disease, cracked tooth, tooth fillings and teeth bleaching can all lead to sensitive teeth.

Movement – there is a natural tooth movement that occurs throughout your life. It could be due to a tooth that is about to fall out, trauma, advanced gum disease or, if you are missing a tooth, the teeth on either side can move to fill in that space.

Discolouration – an indication of a poor diet, or caused by coffee, soft drinks, tobacco, poor dental hygiene, disease, medication, trauma, advanced ageing or using the wrong toothpaste.

GUMS

Pain – this could be due to an injury, dental disease, tooth decay, scurvy, vitamin B deficiency, iron deficiency, Behçet's or Reiter's Syndrome.

Swelling – could be an indication of gum infection, monilia, oral fungal infection, gum disease, gingivitis, poorly fitted dentures, toothpaste or mouthwash allergies. It could also be a possible sign of malnutrition.

Bleeding – this could be due to trauma, disease, mouth sores, systemic conditions, pregnancy and hormonal changes, medication, and vitamin C and K deficiencies.

LIPS

Dry and cracked lips could be caused by external factors such as cold weather, or may be a symptom of dehydration or a nutritional deficiency.

Week 1

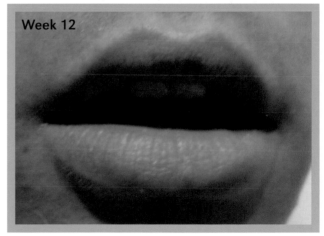

Week 12

You can see that in week 1 I had dry and slightly cracked lips, but by week 12 I had supple and smooth lips thanks to my new diet and using lip balm.

EYES

Your eyes are a big give-away and say a lot about you, how you are feeling, and ultimately how healthy you are. As an organ, the eyes are a great source of information for detecting those early signs of ill

Week 12

due to windy, dry or hot air, or air conditioning. A sluggish thyroid, constant contact lens usage, a deficiency in omega-3 and omega-6, or a reaction to prescriptive and non-prescriptive drugs can also cause dry eyes.

Watery eyes – too many tears being produced could be linked to allergies, a deficiency in vitamin B2 or ocular rosacea.

*Bags under the eye*s – puffy pouches of skin under the eye. This is common as the skin around the eye ages and loses elasticity. Depression, insomnia or deprived sleep, crying, a high level of salt intake, a sluggish thyroid, fluid retention, kidney problems, or a bad reaction to medicine can encourage bags under the eye area.

Circles under the eyes – these could be indications of sleep deprivation, digestive problems, a sluggish liver, eczema or allergies.

Bulging eyes – possibly due to an overactive thyroid. It is important to visit your doctor if you suspect this.

Yellowish lump/bump on the cornea – if you notice these small yellow lumps, don't worry, they tend to be age spots called pinguecula.

Spots on the eye – red spots on the whites of your eyes are usually blood vessels that have burst. It is normally caused by forceful sneezing or coughing, high blood pressure or injury.

health. This is why your doctor will still occasionally examine your eyes when you visit.

Our eyes have more than two million working parts, which make them the second most complex organ in your body (the first is the brain), and while some say eyes are the windows to the soul others have a more practical view.

Red and/or bloodshot – small blood vessels in the eyes become inflamed and dilated which causes bloodshot eyes. This may be caused by, or is an indication of, eye-strain, fatigue, colds, allergies, ocular rosacea, or a deficiency in vitamins B2 and B6 and amino acids commonly found in protein.

It is important to seek medical advice if you are suffering from bloodshot eyes along with any of these symptoms: severe headache, blurred vision, mental confusion, nausea/vomiting, or if you are seeing halos around lights. This may be an indication of an attack of acute glaucoma (a sudden increase in eye pressure).

Yellow eye – if the whites of your eyes turn yellow it could be a possible indication of a liver problem such as jaundice, gallbladder concerns, Gilbert's syndrome, sickle cell anaemia, pancreatic cancer or yellow fever.

Dry eyes – this condition occurs when the eyes don't produce enough tears to keep them moist. It is very common in women, especially after the menopause, due to the body's reduction of the oestrogen hormone.

This could also be environmental, for example,

NAILS

Your fingernails and toenails actually count as part of your skin, and are another great way of highlighting a number of medical and nutritional conditions. Nails are made of protein (keratin) and contain less water than skin, which makes them harder and protects the ends of the fingers and toes.

Fingernails take around four months to grow out, while toenails take at least six. If your nail growth is slower than average, it is possible that you have a fungal infection or a nutritional deficiency such as a lack of iron.

Healthy nails have the following characteristics:

- *Texture* – smooth, no ridges, thickness or cracks
- *Shape* – no exaggerated curving up or down at the ends

- *Nail bed colour* – pink
- *Colour of nails* – white

Here are some things to look out for when investigating your nails.

TEXTURE

Horizontal ridges – these go from side to side across your nail and can be an indication of a thyroid concern, stress, vitamin B deficiency, or the result of a nail injury that has stunted nail growth.

Vertical ridges – these go from the nail bed up to the tip. They may be due to nutritional disorders, a lack of iron, or a kidney disorder.

Pitted nails – this could be caused by lack of vitamin C, psoriasis, or deficiency in protein, and is a common sign for autoimmune disorders.

Thick nails – this could be a result of poor circulation, injury, fungal infection, poor diet or diabetes.

Rough nails – if they have a sandpaper-like texture, rough nails could indicate a skin or hair disorder such as psoriasis or eczema.

Brittle or cracked nails – often this is due to the use of harsh cleaning products, a thyroid disease, iron deficiency, vitamin A deficiency, or a lack of calcium.

Looking at my thumbnail from week 1, you will notice that I have vertical ridges across the nail and a horizontal ridge at the top. This indicates nutritional deficiency.

SHAPE

Nails curve upwards (resembles a spoon) – could be a possible nutritional deficiency, a lack of iron, or a vitamin B12 deficiency.

Nails curve downwards (clubbed nails) – could be an indication of bowel disease, liver disease, or a lack of oxygen in the body. Once this condition occurs, it is normally permanent.

NAIL BED COLOUR

Blue – may be caused by a lung disorder.

Yellow – sign of a heavy smoker, jaundice, or yellow nail syndrome (this is a rare condition however).

Pale – possible sign of anaemia.

White spots – may be due to nail separation from the nail bed, nail warts, zinc or calcium deficiency, or systematic conditions that affect the skin, lungs and other organs.

HAIR AND SCALP

Our hair defines the overall health of a person like no other part of the body. You could say that our luscious locks are a barometer of our general health. Hair condition is a true reflection of the nutrition it receives from the scalp – so the better the diet, the better the hair condition.

Hair is made up from protein (keratin) and minerals, which go through the hair growth cycle. The hair has a growth phase, followed by a resting phase, and then a shedding phase. It then repeats the cycle. When we look at hair, we are looking at its condition, texture and volume to gauge how well our bodies are nourished.

Here are some things to look out for when investigating your hair.

CONDITION

Dry scalp – this could be due to the environment, hard water, poor diet, or the improper use of hair products.

Flaky scalp/dandruff – dandruff is not contagious and is not usually a serious problem. Some cases of excessive dandruff with intense itching and patches of flaky skin elsewhere on your body are most likely to be a form of eczema.

A flaky scalp may be caused by, or is an indication of, a fungus (malassezia), hormone changes, stress, neurological disorders, infrequent shampooing, skin ailments (psoriasis or infections), or the improper use of hair products.

Brittle and split ends – could be due to the environment, a poor diet, lack of protein and essential fatty acids, thyroid disease, menopause, excessive washing and drying, using bleaching and dying products, iodine deficiency, pregnancy, or the improper use of hair products.

VOLUME

Thinning hair/hair loss – this is normally determined by our genes and the ageing process, but may also be caused by a poor diet, lack of iron, or possible thyroid disease.

TEXTURE

Dry – this can be an indication of a poor diet, the environment, lack of protein and essential fatty acids, thyroid disease, menopause, excessive washing and drying, using bleaching and dying products, iodine deficiency, pregnancy, or the improper use of hair products.

Greasy/oily – occurs due to an overproduction of sebum, a waxy substance from the sebaceous glands, which keeps the hair supple, soft and waterproof. Fine hair tends to be greasier due to having more sebaceous glands. It may also be caused by genetics, the improper use of hair products, or a lack of regular hair cleaning.

SKIN

Our skin is a reliable indicator for assessing general health, as it is quite obvious when a person is run down, tired or ill by simply looking at their skin. Just think of all those skin creams and serums produced and marketed to millions of people across the world, claiming to dispel aged or tired looking skin. A good routine and a healthy balance is the basis for picture-perfect skin.

Our skin protects us from the environment, provides a unique barrier to infection, and helps excrete waste and toxins from within the body. It

Look closely, and in the picture on the left you will see a breakout on my chest. But in the next you can see an amazing difference in my skin condition and physique.

regulates and maintains a healthy balance of fluids and minerals, and is of course the source of our sensory receptors for touch. It is the largest organ of the body, and is indirectly linked to almost every part of your body, except the eyes and teeth.

Here are some things to look out for when investigating your skin.

COLOUR

Pale – could be an indication of anaemia or iron deficiency.

Blue tone – may be caused by oxygen deficiency in the blood, exposure to cold temperature, lung disease or heart disease.

Yellow tone – could be jaundice, the consumption of too much beta-carotene (foods such as carrots), or too much vitamin A.

Grey tone – can be caused by excessive smoking, a sluggish liver, cardiovascular disease or feeling unwell.

Red tone – rosacea, over-exertion, inflammation or burns can contribute to a red skin tone. Caught in the early stages, rosacea may cause flushing or blushing, but can progress to permanent redness. The rash consists of tiny pimples as well as dilated blood vessels under the skin and may be found on the face and body, which can cause an itching and burning sensation.

TEXTURE

Dark patches on the skin – possible indication of diabetes and insulin resistance, a hormonal disorder, or an adrenal gland concern.

Scaly rash – can be an indication of psoriasis, an infection or emotional stress.

It is common to find random lumps and bumps either on top of or beneath the skin surface from time to time, and most of these are harmless. Some however are not. If you notice a change in the size or shape of a lump or bump do not hesitate to see your doctor. Early detection of any pre-cancerous or cancerous cells will help treatment. Listen to your body.

FACIAL SKIN

We get oily and dry skin on both our body and face. Here are some things to look out for when investigating your facial skin more closely.

COLOUR

Rosy cheeks – these can be due to a hot flush, overexertion, rosacea, sun damage, or an auto-immune inflammation disease.

Dark patches – these can result from pregnancy, sun damage, a reaction to medication or contraceptive pills, or indicate high levels of oestrogen.

TEXTURE

Oily/greasy – caused by overproduction of sebum, a waxy substance from the sebaceous glands. This could be an indication of stress, pregnancy, hormone imbalance, medication, genetics, or poor diet (high intake of sodium, sugar and saturated fat). The improper use of cosmetic products or a deficiency in vitamin B2 could also cause an outbreak. It is not all bad news, however, your natural sebum slows down the signs of ageing.

It is important to highlight the difference between dry skin and dehydrated skin.

Week 1

Week 12

Look at the amazing difference 12 weeks can make to your skin with the right nutrition, cosmetics and advice.

Dry skin – this lacks the oils and moisture needed to keep skin supple and regulated. If your face never shows an oily shine and you've never even had a pimple (let alone acne), you are most likely to have normal to dry skin. Dry skin may be caused by genetics, or you may be deficient in essential fatty acids (omega-3, omega-6 and omega-9) and/or vitamins A and B. Hormones, skin disorders such as eczema, the environment, and the improper use of cosmetic products could also dry your skin.

Dehydrated skin – this is caused by a lack of water within the cells of the skin. If you have had visible pores, especially around your chin, nose or eyebrows and are prone to spots, but your skin has a dry and scaly appearance, you probably have dehydrated skin. It could be due to dehydration throughout your body, skin disorders (eczema), the improper use of cosmetic products or the environment.

Combination skin – this is characterised by oily patches in certain areas and dry/dehydrated areas in other parts of your face. The normal areas for the oily patch are known as the T-zone: the forehead, nose, cheeks and chin. This is due to these areas having more sebaceous glands than other areas of the face, like the eyes and jaw line. With this combination skin type, awareness must be given to the cosmetic products that you use so that you do not aggravate the problem areas further.

Sensitive skin – thin or fine-textured skin reacts quickly to hot and cold temperatures, and so is easily affected by the environment (sun burn and wind chills). This skin type is usually dry and delicate, and is prone to allergic reactions. Again, awareness must be given to the cosmetic products you use so as to not irritate the skin.

SKIN CARE ROUTINE

There are a lot of things you can do to keep your skin healthy, feeling fresh, soft and looking young. Maintaining a healthy diet, getting enough exercise, staying hydrated, avoiding any sun damage to the skin, and having low stress levels are all things that aid in keeping skin healthy. Following a skin care routine can also help. The skin care cycle has three main steps that should be followed daily to ensure a truly glowing complexion.

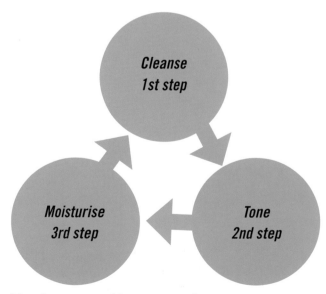

The three step skin care routine.

What is cleansing?

Throughout the day your skin is exposed to all kinds of things that clog up your pores, such as exhaust fumes, pollution, bacteria and dirt. Your skin naturally looses dead cells, excretes sweat (laced with toxins that your body is pushing out) and excess sebum.

By the end of the day, all this grime lies on the top of the skin and needs removing. When you cleanse, you remove this build-up. Oil-based, clay and scrub cleansers will also remove the top layer of dead skin.

What is toning?

This step is so simple and so often overlooked. Ultimately it is crucial to balance the skin, add nutrients and increase hydration. Toning removes any remaining grime left by the cleanser (which is especially important with oil-based cleansers), and will balance the pH of the skin. It will also aid in the tightening of pores, and helps the skin absorb oils more effectively.

What is moisturising?

This is the most important step in the cycle, and helps keep skin young and soft. Think about a piece of leather, for example. Adding oil keeps it from drying out, losing vibrancy and wrinkling. Cleansing removes the skin's natural oils on dry skin, on oily skin it signals to the skin to stimulate more oil production often causing overproduction. By not replacing these oils, the skin must work harder to balance itself.

A moisturiser is not just oil, though – it should be a blend of good quality ingredients, as it sinks into the skin. Using a cheaper alternative often means cheaper ingredients that will have a long-term negative effect on the skin's appearance.

LOOKING AFTER YOUR BODY

With all of the information you have just gained, you may now be wondering what you can do to help yourself.

One thing you may have noticed is that poor nutrition– lacking in vitamins and minerals – plays an important role in giving signs of poor health. By changing the way you eat, and by choosing a rounded diet that is nutritious and high in vitamins and minerals, your body will return to full health.

For any health concerns that you may have, you can help yourself in many ways, ranging from homeopathic remedies and supplements to holistic therapies. Whatever concerns you may have, remember there is nothing too big or too small for your GP. They are there to help you.

TAKE CONTROL OF THE BASICS

When we look at the basics for health, we are looking at the situations that we face every day of our lives. How we handle stress, how we overcome tiredness, and how we get the most out of ourselves.

It is these situations that change the way we look at life and make us into who we are. If we can take hold of these basics, we will be able to get more out of ourselves and others.

STRESS

We feel stress when pressure is placed upon us, whether actual or imagined. It can be harmful, but a certain amount can be good for us to help motivation, performance and productivity. Too much stress, however, can prompt depression, so please keep a close eye on yourself and others.

People react differently to stress; some have a higher threshold than others. Reasons for stress are very broad and unpredictable. It is a common fact that stress can be caused by demanding deadlines at work, the loss of a loved one, relationship concerns, financial pressures or illness. These and many more concerns can cause anxiety and stress, which can lead to physical, emotional and mental health problems. When we are faced with circumstances that are stressful to our mind and body, the body releases hormones (chemicals like cortisol and adrenaline), which help regulate our responses internally.

Adrenaline, for instance, is released to help us cope with dangerous or unexpected conditions. These invoke the 'flight or fight' impulse – the biological response to acute stress. It is interesting, however, that when faced with a situation in which you are prevented from either fleeing or fighting,

such as being in a crowded underground station, these chemicals are not released. If you have a build-up of these chemicals due to them not being used the consequences are felt throughout the body, such as an increase in blood pressure, heart rate and sweat production.

Stress can cause single or multiple conditions. The list below is not meant to scare you, it is simply to emphasise the need to try to control and minimise any stress you may feel in your life:

- Heart disease
- Muscular tension
- Pain
- Diet
- Depression
- Weight gain/loss/obesity
- Digestive problems
- Sleep problems
- Autoimmune diseases
- Lower immunity causing more colds, feeling run down, etc.
- Raised cholesterol
- Skin complaints

STRESS RESPONSES

Stress affects our bodies in many ways and on many levels. Have a look below to understand your stress responses.

- *Physiological* – tension from posture or overuse.
- *Emotional* – anger, fear and hate are all reflected in our postures.
- *Behavioural* – posture imbalance from habit.
- *Structural* – the body and posture will change to meet any stress imposed upon it.

You can follow these steps to help control your own stress levels.

Step 1 – your stress levels

These are influenced by numerous things. The key is to have the knowledge and power to monitor your own responses, and to seek help or advice when something gets a little too much for you to cope with. How you take control is up to you.

Step 2 – your sense of control

Have confidence in yourself and your ability to perform. Support from friends and family will encourage you to look on the positive side and to share some of your concerns, and will act as a buffer for life's stresses, resulting in you feeling less vulnerable.

Step 3 – your attitude

Try to have a more optimistic outlook. The ability to manage your emotions and bring them back into balance will enable you to become more calm and relaxed.

Step 4 – your understanding and preparation

Learn from past stresses and try to be prepared for similar future stresses. For example, when I broke my back in a diving accident, I knew it would be a long road to recovery so I rehabilitated slowly and professionally trying not to worry excessively about things. I made a full recovery and have continued diving with no worries.

KEEPING TRACK OF STRESS

During the 12-week programme I used the RPE scale to track stress levels. As you can see from the graph, stress levels were fairly high at the start, but gradually decreased by eating healthily, exercising and taking control of my body's condition and lifestyle. The male results in the table are my results during the 12-week programme.

RPE (RATING PERCEIVED EXERTION)

The RPE scale is a simple method of measuring how a person handles stress on their body. The original scale was introduced by Gunnar Borg, who rated exertion on a scale of 6–20, although many health practitioners now use a revised scale of 0–10, developed by the American College of Sports Medicine. RPE can be applied to absolutely anything:

0 Not stressed at all
1 Very, very light stress
2 Very light stress
3 Fairly light stress
4 Light amount of stress
5 Moderately stressed
6 Fairly stressed
7 Stressed
8 Very stressed
9 Very, very stressed
10 Stress is severely affecting life

ENERGY LEVELS

It's a fact: having more energy in the body fights fatigue and reduces stress levels. We have all felt tired and lacking in energy from time to time, especially during busy or stressful periods. But if you know the cause then the solution is often easy. More often than not, the reasons are found in our everyday life and habits.

Energy levels can be affected by your diet, how much sleep you get, and even your emotional state. There are many contributing factors that affect the balance of our emotional and physical state, which ultimately affect our energy levels. You should ask yourself how many of the following items are you managing to help keep your batteries charged:

- Having regular exercise
- Drinking plenty of water
- Eating a balanced diet
- Sleeping well
- Controlling stress levels
- Managing your emotional state

KEEPING TRACK OF TIREDNESS LEVELS

During the 12-week programme, use the RPE scale to track your progress in overcoming tiredness. We changed the stress scale to a tiredness rating:

0 Not tired at all
1 Very, very samll amount of tiredness
2 Very small amount of tiredness
3 Fairly small amount of tiredness
4 Small amount of tiredness
5 Moderately tired
6 Fairly tired

7 Tired
8 Very tired
9 Very, very tired
10 Too tired to stay awake

The results show how I was handling my energy levels on a daily basis. As you can see, my tiredness levels were fairly high at the start of the 12 weeks, but gradually decreased as I started to eat healthily,

Stress level results

Tiredness level results

This is me running the bleep test on week 4. I never really like doing this test, but it has to be done to see how well training is going.

exercise and basically gain control of my body and its condition. Although I did suffer from a fair amount of tiredness, I was able to manage it by following the steps above.

SLEEP

Sleep is as important as eating and drinking, which is why we spend one third of our lives doing it. It is absolutely vital for maintaining a normal level of cognitive skills, including speech, memory, and innovative and flexible thinking, and it gives the body a chance to recuperate and recover from all of the day's activities.

We all become agitated and stressed when we are tired. The most simple and mundane tasks may become a source of stress due to sleep deprivation. Most adults need to sleep for around eight hours a night on a regular basis to function well, although some require more than others. It is believed the likes of Napoleon, Florence Nightingale and Margaret Thatcher all survived on just four hours sleep a night.

Sleep is triggered by hormones that are active in the brain, and respond to cues from the body and the environment. Some of our growth hormones trigger the release of proteins throughout the body to build and repair cells during sleep. Sleep deprivation can prevent this and affect the immune system.

Sleep occurs in a recurrent series of 90–110 minute bursts, and is divided into two categories relating to eye movement levels: REM (rapid eye movement) sleep, and non-REM sleep, which is about 80 per cent of all sleep.

During non-REM sleep, your breathing and heart rate slow and blood pressure will be low. This type of sleep is divided into four stages:

Level 1 transition between wakefulness to sleep
Level 2 makes up 50 per cent of sleep, slowing breathing and heartbeat
Level 3 very low respiration and heartbeat
Level 4 leads to rapid eye movement sleep known as REM, or Level 5

My average amount of sleep per night was six hours, 36 minutes, while my female counterpart slept on average seven hours and five minutes per night.

HYDRATION

Water makes up more than two thirds of the weight of the human body, around 60–70 per cent depending on size, shape and the amount of lean tissue (muscle). Muscle consists of approximately 75 per cent water, fat is around 14 per cent, blood has around 82 per cent, and lungs have 90 per cent. Astonishingly, the human brain is made up of 95 per cent water. A mere 2per cent drop in our body's water supply can trigger signs of dehydration, and without water we would die within days.

Water is the most important nutrient for the body. It helps keep your cells, tissues and organs running smoothly, efficiently and effectively. Some of the ways water keeps your body working is by helping to keep it at a constant internal temperature, preventing constipation, and by cushioning your joints and protecting your organs. Fluids are vitally important when you are ill, particularly when you lose more water due to fever, diarrhoea or vomiting.

Your body needs a continuous supply of water to stay hydrated. By maintaining an adequate hydration level, your body will feel all the more healthy.

Reasons why water is special:

- Helps to fight fatigue and tiredness
- Allows you to exercise, train harder and maintain your strength
- Is the best detoxing agent available
- Helps digestion
- Regulates your metabolism
- Serves as a lubricant
- Forms the base for saliva
- Forms fluids that surround and protect joints
- Regulates the body temperature as cooling and heating is distributed through perspiration
- Helps get rid of waste

If you always wait until your mouth is dry to drink water, then you are probably waiting too long and are likely to be dehydrated. Dehydration causes a fuzzy short-term memory, trouble with basic cognitive skills and difficulty focusing on smaller print. Are you having trouble reading this? If so, drink up.

Water comes packaged in different forms, so you can have a little variety throughout your day. Did you know that a glass of milk or a serving of juice is actually about 90 per cent water? Some foods have high water content too, such as fruits, vegetables, yoghurts and soups. Enjoying these foods regularly can contribute to your water intake, and also provide you with many of the vitamins and minerals your body needs.

Here's something to think about: a common mistake is confusing thirst for hunger, so why not drink water if you feel hungry between meals?

How much water is enough? It is recommended that we consume between 1.5 and 3 litres a day. During the 12-week programme I drank 1.5 litres a day (eight glasses) on average, and that's excluding the fruit drinks, herbal teas and food I consumed. Don't be put off by plain water. Add cordial to it to make it a little tastier.

POSTURE

Posture plays such an important role in the health of your body, but more often than not it is simply overlooked. The ideal skeletal alignment and consequent good posture involves teaching your body to stand, lie, walk and sit in positions that require the least amount of strain on supporting ligaments during any bodily movement. Having good posture keeps bones and joints in the correct alignment so that muscles are used correctly. It prevents fatigue because muscles are being used more effectively and therefore using less energy, and even contributes to a good appearance – more supermodel, less hunchback.

ANALYSING YOUR POSTURE

Your posture provides a lot of information about the state of your body. Postural analysis allows you to see which areas of the body are under more stress than others, which could result in the kind of backache that I was experiencing before starting the 12-week programme.

The easiest way to see if you have a good posture is to stand next to a plumb line to see if any body parts are out of sync. I use this method on clients to identify any postural faults and to help to distinguish which areas I need to strengthen or release. The side view posture test hypothetically divides the body into front and back sections of equal weight.

During the 12-week programme, you should take photos of your posture from the side and front to see the improvements in your posture. This method is not as accurate as if you were to visit a health professional, but it is something that can be done at home. Please note, you will need someone to help you with this test.

Set-up
Postural alignment equipment:

- Plain wall
- Plumb bob and line (coloured string if possible, available from most DIY stores)
- Picture hook
- Tape measure
- Camera

Tie the plumb line string to a picture hook in the ceiling in front of the wall you are going to stand in front of.

Standing barefoot, ensure the plumb line passes slightly forward of the ankle and approximately through the apex of the arch of the foot.

Then measure the distance between the wall and your feet, as well as between your feet themselves, and use these measurements to ensure you are positioned in the same way every four weeks when you take photos of your posture.

Analyse, compare and diagnose your own posture against that of a neutral posture using the following guidelines and pictures. If you have a misaligned posture then use the information given here to strengthen or stretch your muscles to realign yourself.

NEUTRAL POSTURE

In the neutral position, all the muscles are working in harmony with each other, and there are no elongated, weak, or short and strong muscles.

Week 1   Week 4   Week 8   Week 12

These photos show you the transformation that your body will undergo through 12 weeks. It is amazing how, with the right training, stretching and nutrition routines, and with a little help from the myo massage, your posture can be corrected.

If a person with a neutral posture stands side on, the plumb line should pass through the following areas:

- Head: lobe of the ear.
- Cervical spine: the neck presents a normal anterior curve.
- Thoracic: the thoracic spine should curve slightly in a posterior direction, and the plumb line should pass midway through the shoulder joint.

- Lumbar: the lumbar should curve slightly anterior.
- Pelvis: the front (anterior) and the back (posterior) of your hip should be at the same angle.
- Hip joint: slightly posterior to the centre of the hip.
- Knee: slightly anterior through the axis of the knee joint. The knee should be neither flexed nor extended.
- Ankle: past the ankle and through the apex of the arch of the foot.
- Feet.

Neutral

Lordotic

Kyphotic

Flat back

Strong muscles
Elongated muscles

Sway back

C shape

Your feet should be in a neutral position, with your toes angled outward slightly at approximately 8 to 10°, and your heels together.

There are five common misaligned posture types illustrated on this page and detailed in the table overleaf.

	Kyphotic posture	Lordotic posture	Flat back posture	Sway back posture	C-shape posture
Key features	Rounded and elongated upper back	Bigger arch in lower back	No or limited arch in lower back	Long curve from upper back to lower back; pelvis, spine and shoulders tilt slightly towards one side	Shoulder lower on same side as raised hip with curvature dependent on muscle strength and weakness
Head	Forward	Neutral	Forward	Forward	Normal/neutral
Cervical spine	Hyper-extended	Normal/neutral (slight anterior)	Slightly extended (causes head to tilt up)	Slightly extended (causes head to tilt up)	Normal/neutral
Shoulder					Elevated, adducted or slightly depressed (raised up, in or down)
Thoracic spine	Increased flexion (increased posterior curve/rounded shoulders)	Normal/neutral (slight posterior)	Increased flexion at top, straightens towards bottom (round shoulders into a straight lower back)	Increased flexion (long kyphosis)	Slight curvature either to left or right
Lumbar	Neutral	Hyper-extended (greater curve in lower back)	Hyper-flexed (lower back becomes straight)	Flexion (flattening of lower back)	Slight curvature either to left or right
Pelvis	Neutral	Anterior tilt (tilts down forwards)	Posterior tilt (backwards/up)	Posterior tilt (backwards/up)	Lateral tilt on left or right
Hip joint	Flexed	Flexed	Extended	Hyper-extended	Adducted and slightly medial rotated on one side (one side forward and in/down and other up)
Knee	Normal/neutral	Slightly hyper-extended	Slightly hyper-extended	Slightly hyper-extended	
Ankle	Normal/neutral	Slight plantar flexion (toes point down towards floor as body leans on toes)	Normal/neutral	Slight plantar flexion (toes point down towards floor as body leans on toes)	

	Elongated or weak muscles	Exercises to strengthen muscles	Short or strong muscles	Exercises to stretch muscles
Kyphotic posture	Neck flexors, upper back, external obliques, and hamstrings (slightly elongated but may or may not be weak)	• Reverse shrugs • Bent-over lat raises • T-bar row	Neck extensors and possibly your pectorals	Static stretch for the chest on a wall trapezius stretch Static stretch for the trapezius muscles
Lordotic posture	Abdominals and hamstrings may or may not be elongated	• Reverse curl • Reverse crunch • Stiff leg deadlifts	Lower back and hip flexor/rectus femoris	PNF stretch for quad lying face down Developmental stretch for the lower back while lying down Developmental stretch for hip flexor stretch
Flat back posture	Hip flexors and the back may seem elongated with a flat back, but they may not be weak	• Reverse crunch • Deadlifts • Dorsal raises	Hamstrings and the abdominals are frequently strong	PNF stretch for hamstring muscles Developmental stretch for sitting hamstring muscles Static stretch for the abdominal muscles
Sway back posture	Hip joint flexors, external oblique, upper back extensors and neck extensors	• Bent-over row • Single arm cable row	Hamstrings and the upper part of the internal oblique; lower back is normally strong but not short	Developmental stretch for sitting hamstring muscles PNF stretch for hamstring muscles
C-shape posture	Lateral trunk muscles, the hip adductors (inside thigh), inside of calf muscles, and on the opposite side the hip abductors (gluteus medius muscle), and also TFL (front of hip) – side where pelvis tilts lower is weak side		Hamstrings and abdominals are often strong. For instance, the hip/pelvis that is raised/tilted up has tight lateral muscles, hip adductors (inside thigh), inside calf muscles, and on the opposite side the abductors (gluteus medius muscle). Also look at the TFL (front of hip). Strong muscles are opposite side to weak muscles.	

Scoliosis

Strong muscles
Elongated muscles

UNDERSTANDING AND TESTING YOUR BODY'S HEALTH

In order to monitor your progress and to demonstrate your eventual results, you should take health tests before, during and after the 12-week fitness and nutrition programme. We've opted for home testing instead of visiting a GP every week. These tests are not as accurate as those you may receive from your doctor, so perhaps visit your GP before and after your 12-week programme. This will ensure both sets of your results are accurate, and if you do have any health concerns before you start the programme, your doctor will be able to advise you.

Most of the home health-testing kits are easily available at a pharmacy or online.

Equipment needed for the health tests:

- Accurate scales
- Tape measure
- Glucose home test
- Cholesterol home test
- Callipers
- Body fat percentage reader
- Peak flow meter
- Watch
- Blood pressure monitor

Scoliosis

An S-shape posture, where the shoulder is raised higher on the same side as a raised hip, could be scoliosis. Scoliosis is the abnormal curvature of the spine to the sides, which should be diagnosed by a doctor observing the movement in your back.

HELP TO REALIGN YOUR POSTURE

Now you can identify which category your posture falls into, you can take the correct steps to amend it by strengthening and shortening the weak muscles with exercise, and by elongating the short, strong muscles by stretching them. Exercises and stretches found within the 12-week programme can help with realigning posture, and massage can also help to alleviate muscular tension.

Blood pressure monitor

Each of the following tests was taken at the start of the programme, with some repeated on the last day of each week, and all taken every four weeks.

Tests	Every week	Every 4 weeks
Height and weight	x	x
BMI	x	x
Resting heart rate (RHR)	x	x
Blood pressure (BP)	x	x
Body fat percentage	x	x
Measurements	x	x
Glucose		x
Cholesterol		x
Lung function		x
Calliper tests		x

HEIGHT AND WEIGHT

Although your height will give you no relevant information on its own, apart from telling you how tall or (in my case) how short you are, you will need it in order to work out your BMI.

Jumping on the scales every day is not the most accurate way to follow your progress, and try not to put too much pressure on yourself to lose a specific amount of weight each week. Don't weigh yourself every day, as this can be very disheartening, but do it every Sunday on test day. You will need to weigh yourself to work out your BMI.

Body mass index (BMI)

There is no average weight or size that a person should be, but there is a method to discover if we fit into the general health practitioners' recommendations. Using height and weight measurements we can use the BMI to determine a healthy weight for your height.

For the 12-week programme, we used a body fat percentage monitor for calculating BMI, but you can use the BMI equation below to calculate it if you don't have one. It is a quick and effective technique to work out the weight range you are in:

$$\text{Weight (kg)} \div \text{height (m)} = x$$
$$x \div \text{height (m)} = \text{BMI}$$

For example, if you weigh 80kg and you are 1.75m tall, your BMI would be 26.1 (80 ÷ 1.75 = 45.7, then 45.7 ÷ 1.75 = 26.1). Using the chart below, you can see that the end figure would mean that the person is overweight. Please note, however, that BMI should not be used by bodybuilders or athletes as they have a higher than normal amount of muscle mass.

The BMI chart

Underweight	13–18
Normal weight	19–24
Overweight	25–29
Obese/seriously overweight	30–40
Dangerously overweight/morbidly obese	40+

RESTING HEART RATE (RHR)

This test measures your heart's efficiency in pumping blood around the body when you are in a resting state. The RHR is able to tell you how fit you are, and by following the 12-week programme you should see a steady decrease in your heart rate as your heart becomes more efficient. Try and take your RHR readings as soon as you wake up in the morning, to get your best record.

You can find your RHR by simply finding your pulse on the thumb side of the wrist, and counting your heartbeat for one minute with your index and middle finger to see what result you have.

At the beginning of week 1 my RHR was 79 beats per minute, and by the end of week 12 it had decreased to 37 beats per minute.

The table overleaf shows the average RHR for a male. Mark where you are on the table to see how fit you are right now, and then mark it again in 12 weeks' time.

Resting heart rate for men

Age	18–25	26–35	36–45	46–55	56–65	65+
Athlete	<55	<54	<56	<57	<56	<55
Excellent	56–61	55–61	57–62	58–63	57–61	56–61
Good	62–65	62–65	63–66	64–67	62–67	62–65
Fair	66–69	66–70	67–70	68–71	68–71	66–69
Average	70–73	71–74	71–75	72–76	72–75	70–73
Poor	74–81	75–81	76–82	77–83	76–81	74–79
Very poor	82+	82+	83+	84+	82+	80+

This is a blood pressure monitor similar to the one used in the 12-week programme.

BLOOD PRESSURE

Checking blood pressure is essential, as it directly affects your health. Blood pressure testing measures the strength of your heartbeat and the pressure of the circulating blood against the walls of your blood vessels. An ideal, healthy blood pressure is 120 over 80. The first number is your systolic blood pressure (the highest pressure when your heart beats), and the second number is your diastolic blood pressure (the lowest pressure when your heart relaxes between beats).

	Systolic	Diastolic
Low	70–90	40–60
Ideal	90–120	60–80
Pre-high	120–140	80–90
High	140–190+	90–100+

My blood pressure was at 130/92 in week 1, and after completing the 12-week programme it was 127/44.

BODY FAT PERCENTAGE

This is a quicker and more convenient version of the calliper test. However, the results are not quite as accurate. If you do this test every week it will allow you to see the change and will keep you on track.

There are a number of body fat monitor models available; some are similar to normal bathroom scales that you stand on with bare feet, others are hand-held. The monitor passes a low-level, imperceptible electric current through your body.

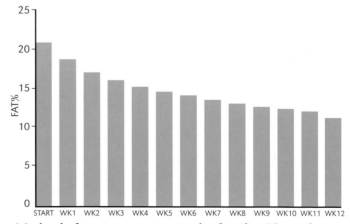

My body fat percentage results for the 12-week programme.

Fat contains limited water and is not a good conductor, so it impedes the current. As lean body tissue contains mainly water and electrolytes, this conducts the current throughout the body giving you a reading. By measuring your lean body mass, the monitor can predict your fat mass.

For best results, the monitors should be used at the same time of day, once a week, with minimal clothing being worn. You will also need to empty your bladder before use, as this will affect the results. Also, avoid alcohol and use the device straight after exercising.

MEASUREMENTS

I use measurements constantly with clients, as well as in my own training, as it is a great way to show how the body is reacting to your exercise and nutrition. With the results of your measurements and your fat percentage, you will be able to see if you are losing body fat rather than just losing weight (which may well just be fluid).

To take measurements accurately, you will need someone else to take them for you so your body can relax in a standing position. Take measurements while cold and relaxed, and at the same time every week throughout the 12-week programme. Please take careful note of exactly where you are taking your measurements from, and ensure that you measure from exactly the same place every time, in order to keep your results as precise as possible.

- Neck: measure down from where the ear lobe and jaw connect. The measurement will be down to the largest part of the neck. Take a note of the measurement, and then measure around the neck for the result.
- Chest: place the tape measure around the upper torso, measuring from the nipples and keeping the tape in the same alignment all of the way around.
- Upper arm: look at the arm and mark out the largest circumference. Measure up from the lateral epicondyle of the humerus (the bony bit on the outside of the elbow). Take note of the measurement, and then measure around the circumference for the result. Repeat for the opposite arm.

Week 4

Week 12

Not bad in just 8 weeks, a gain of 1½ inches.

- Waist/naval: place the tape measure around your abdomen, measuring from the belly button and keeping the tape in alignment all the way around.
- Hips: place the tape measure around the hips over the anterior superior iliac spine (or the bony parts either side of your hip). Make sure the tape goes all of the way around and is in alignment with the front.
- Upper thigh: look at the widest part on the upper thigh and mark. Measure up from the head of the fibula (or the bony part on the outside of the top of the lower leg). Take note of the measurement,

Week 4

Week 12

I lost a lot of inches from my waist, but this was not all body weight.

and then measure around the circumference for the result. Repeat for the opposite thigh.

- Calf: look at the largest part on the calf and measure around its circumference. Repeat for the opposite calf.

GLUCOSE TEST

This test measures the amount of glucose in the blood, and is used to detect hyperglycaemia (higher than normal glucose levels in the blood) and hypoglycaemia (lower than normal glucose levels in the blood). It also helps identify diabetes.

For the tests, we used a fasting blood glucose test for ease, which required eating no later than 10 p.m. the night before and taking the test at around 8 a.m. the following morning. Keeping the test criteria the same provides the best results. Please make sure that you read and follow the instructions on the specific test kit that you use.

The result guidelines for the fasting blood glucose test I took are in the table below, measured in millimoles per litre (mmol/l).

From 3.6 to 6.0 mmol/l	Normal fasting glucose
From 6.1 to 6.9 mmol/l	Impaired fasting glucose
7.0 mmol/l and above	Probable diabetes

CHOLESTEROL TEST

Our bodies need a certain amount of cholesterol to make cell membranes, insulate nerves and produce hormones. Cholesterol is a waxy substance produced in the liver and other organs. We can also absorb cholesterol from foods such as eggs, red meat, cheese and more. Too much or too high a cholesterol level can affect your heart.

There are two forms of cholesterol, one of which is good for you while the other is bad.

Good cholesterol

High-density lipoprotein (HDL) picks up and transports surplus cholesterol from the body tissues back to the liver, where it is broken down and passed out of the body.

Bad cholesterol

Low-density lipoprotein (LDL) transports cholesterol from the liver around the rest of the body. When there is more LDL in the blood than the body needs, the cholesterol accumulates in the body tissues, such as the walls of the coronary arteries. Here it can build-up and affect the heart function.

A home test cholesterol kit

A home test kit simply measures the total amount of cholesterol. Please remember to read and follow the instructions. The levels of total cholesterol fall into the following categories, as shown in the table below.

Ideal level	3.9–5.2 mmol/l
Mildly high level	5.0–6.4 mmol/l
High level	6.5–7.8 mmol/l
Very high level	7.8+ mmol/l

LUNG FUNCTION TEST

The lung function test is measured by a peak flow meter, a small hand-held device used to measure how fast a person can exhale. The peak expiratory flow rate (PEFR) shows how well your airways are performing.

To measure PEFR:

- Breathe in as deeply as possible
- Blow out into the meter as hard and fast as possible
- Take note of its result and repeat three times and record your highest rate

My lung function reading on the peak flow meter increased from 600 to 700 as my fitness improved on the 12-week programme.

Average male lung function results

Age	Height (m)							
	1.55	**1.60**	**1.65**	**1.70**	**1.75**	**1.80**	**1.85**	**1.90**
25	515	534	552	570	589	607	625	644
30	502	520	539	557	576	594	612	632
35	489	508	526	544	563	582	600	619
40	476	495	513	531	550	568	586	606
45	463	482	501	519	537	556	574	593
50	450	469	487	505	524	543	561	580
55	438	456	475	493	511	530	548	567
60	424	443	462	480	498	517	535	545
65	412	430	449	460	486	504	522	541
70	399	417	436	545	472	491	509	528

CALLIPER TEST

This test measures skin folds to calculate your body's fat percentage. You will need to have another person available to help take the measurements for this test, but again this can be done at home.

To take the calliper test

- Use the left-hand side for all of your measurements with your arms hanging freely.
- Pinch 1cm above the area being measured with the calliper.

- Measure all your calliper positions so that the next reading will be taken in the same place.
- The pinch should be maintained throughout the reading for a specific area before moving on towards the next area.
- Take the measurement a couple of times to gain the most accurate reading, allowing the skin to return to normal between readings.

Areas to measure

- Biceps – vertical fold for the pinch. Measure half way between the shoulder and the elbow directly on to the biceps to take the reading.
- Triceps – vertical fold for the pinch. Measure half way between the shoulder and the elbow directly on to the triceps to take the reading.

Calliper

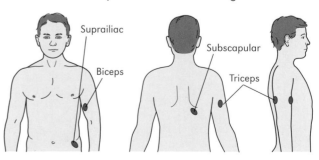

Suprailiac

Biceps

Subscapular

Triceps

- Suprailiac – diagonal fold for the pinch. Measure directly above the hip.
- Subscapular – diagonal fold for the pinch. Measure 1–2cm down at 45° directly from the bottom of the shoulder blade.

Now add all four of your calliper measurements (biceps, triceps, superiliac and subscapular) together to get your total skin folds measurement. Apply your total skin folds measurement to the appropriate tables below:

Average male calliper test results

Total measurements for all four skin folds (mm)	Age 16–29 (fat %)	Age 30–49 (fat %)	Age 50 (fat %)
20	8.1	12.1	12.5
22	9.2	13.2	13.9
24	10.2	14.2	15.1
26	11.2	15.2	16.3
28	12.1	16.1	17.4
30	12.9	16.9	17.5
35	14.7	18.7	20.8
40	16.3	20.3	22.8
45	17.7	21.8	24.7
50	19.0	23.0	26.3
55	20.2	24.2	27.8
60	21.2	25.3	29.1
65	22.2	26.2	30.4
70	23.2	27.1	31.5
75	24.0	28.0	32.6
80	24.8	28.8	33.7
85	25.6	29.6	34.6
90	26.3	30.3	35.5
95	27.0	31.0	36.5
100	27.6	31.7	37.3
110	28.8	32.9	38.8
120	29.9	34.0	40.2
130	31.0	35.0	41.5
140	31.9	36.0	42.8
150	32.8	36.8	43.9
Lean	<10	<13	<14
Optimal	10–15	13–17	14–19
Slightly overweight	16–20	18–22	20–24
Overweight	21–24	23–26	25–27
Obese	>25	>26	>27

HEALTHY EATING

03

KNOWING YOUR FOODS AND FOLLOWING THE PLAN

The meals and recipes in this book are easy to follow, and have been created with a family of four in mind (but do feel free to make smaller amounts for individual portions). It is important to show that following a healthy and balanced nutritional diet will improve you and your family's health, fitness and well-being. The recipe section will guide you through the number of meals that you should consume each day, when and how to prepare them, and even supplies you with detailed weekly shopping lists to save you time.

The shopping lists include all of the ingredients that you will need for each week's recipes, and you can find printable versions online (www.bloomsbury.com/9781408196366), which you can print off and take with you when you go shopping. The lists are divided into sections, from carbohydrates through to meat, fish, fruit and vegetables, and you will find shopping much quicker and easier with them. Please feel free to amend the lists to incorporate your existing cupboard contents. Vegetarians and vegans can substitute tofu, soya or Quorn products for meat, fish and dairy items in recipes.

HEALTHY EATING VERSUS UNHEALTHY EATING

It is never too late to make a difference, and with some changes to your fitness, nutrition and lifestyle you can make big changes, with great results.

STARTING YOUR WEIGHT LOSS

You may be wondering if the nutrition programme is going to work for you. Well, I followed it and look at the great results I got.

By eating a healthy balanced diet your health results should improve, as well as your fitness results. When you get the right nutrition it contributes to around 60–70 per cent of how you look and feel.

If you have mistreated your body, you have the ability to change your health and well-being for the better, as our bodies are great at adapting to new lifestyles and diets.

The best way to start this plan is by emptying the contents of your fridge and cupboards – get rid of all the junk and unhealthy foods. Not only will this give you a fresh start, but it will also stop any temptations further down the line.

KNOWING YOUR FOODS

Foods come in various forms, and have a variety of benefits for our bodies. We have natural foods and processed foods, and here we find out why natural foods are so much more important for us.

Here is a quick rundown of every important type of food group/property that you are likely to come across:

- Carbohydrates – our main source of energy.
- Proteins – essential for growth and repair of muscle and other body tissues.
- Fats – a source of energy and important in relation to fat-soluble vitamins.
- Minerals – these are inorganic elements that occur in our bodies, and which are critical to its normal function.
- Vitamins – water- and fat-soluble vitamins play important roles in many chemical processes in the body.
- Water – essential for our body's healthy functioning. It makes up 60–70 per cent of the human body, and is used to carry nutrients around.

Nutrition affects 60–70% of the way we look.

CARBOHYDRATES (CARBS)

Carbohydrate (meaning 'carbon plus water') is the most widely eaten food in the world. Along with fat and protein, carbohydrate is an essential nutrient, but what makes carbs different is that they are easily converted into energy by the body. Carbohydrates come in two forms – simple and complex.

Simple carbohydrates – various forms of sugar, such as glucose and sucrose (table sugar). These simple carbs have smaller molecules, making it easier for them to be absorbed into the body and used as energy. Fruit, dairy products and honey contain large amounts of simple carbohydrates.

Complex carbohydrates – composed of long-string simple carbs. This means the body absorbs the large molecules at a slower rate than the simpler molecules, which gives us energy at a slower rate than simple carbs, but faster than fats and protein. Complex carbs consist of rice, bread, beans and root vegetables (e.g. potatoes).

Carbohydrates can also be classed as refined or unrefined.

Refined carbohydrates – highly processed products, with all of the goodness such as fibre, bran, vitamins and minerals stripped away, but still giving the same amount of calories.

Refined products often include vitamins and minerals that have been added in an unnatural way, giving the food little nutritional value.

You should reduce or eliminate these types of refined products, such as white bread, white rice, cakes, commercial cereals, biscuits, crisps, bagels and croissants from your diet. If you tend to get most of your carbs from these refined products, you run a higher risk of getting type-2 diabetes and becoming obese.

Unrefined carbohydrates – untouched products still retaining their original nutritional value. Brown rice, wholegrain bread, muesli and yams are all unrefined carbs.

If you consume more carbohydrates than your body needs at any one time, your body stores some of these within cells as glycogen and converts the rest into fat. So remember, only eat what you need to remain satisfied.

PROTEIN

The body needs proteins to maintain and replace tissues, and to function and grow. If the body is getting enough calories, it does not use protein for energy. If more protein is consumed than is needed, the body breaks the protein down and stores its components as fat.

Protein is the main building block in the body, and is the primary component of most cells: muscle, connective tissues, hair and skin are all built from protein.

Protein consists of units called amino acids, strung together in complex formations. Because proteins are complex molecules the body takes longer to break them down. As a result, they are a longer-lasting source of energy than carbohydrates.

Amino acids – the 20 amino acids found in proteins convey a vast array of chemical versatility. The body synthesises some of them from components within the body, but there are nine amino acids that the body cannot synthesise. These are called essential amino acids, and they must be consumed within your diet.

Essential amino acids – adults need eight of these nine amino acids: isoleucine, leucine, lysine, methionine, phenylalanine, threonine, tryptophan and valine. Infants also need a ninth one: histidine.

The percentage of protein the body can use to synthesise essential amino acids varies from protein to protein. The body can use 100 per cent of the protein in an egg, and a high percentage of the proteins in milk and meats.

FATS

Fats are complex molecules composed of fatty acids and glycerol. The body needs fats for growth and energy, and the body also uses them to synthesise hormones and other substances (such as prostaglandins) needed for the body's activities.

Fats are the slowest source of energy, but the most energy efficient form of food. Each gram of fat supplies the body with about nine calories – more than twice that supplied by proteins or carbohydrates.

As fats are such an efficient form of energy, the body stores any excess energy as fat. The body deposits excess fat in the abdomen (omental fat) and under the skin (subcutaneous fat) to use when it needs more energy. The body may also deposit excess fat in blood vessels and within organs, where it can block blood flow and damage organs, often causing serious disorders. The different types of fats are listed below.

Saturated fats – these are more likely to increase cholesterol levels and increase the risk of atherosclerosis. Products containing saturated fats include: meat products (especially beef), coconut and palm oil, as well as artificial hydrogenated fat.

Monounsaturated fats – normally lowers LDL cholesterol (the 'bad' cholesterol), and is found in both plant and animal products, such as olive oil, canola oil and peanut oil, and in some plant foods such as avocado.

Polyunsaturated fats – these tend to lower blood cholesterol levels, and are found in plant sources such as safflower, sunflower, corn and cottonseed, and oils such as olive oil, and walnut oil.

Essential Fatty Acids (EFAs) – these are necessary fats that the human body cannot synthesise, and must be obtained through diet. EFAs are long-chain polyunsaturated fatty acids derived from linolenic, linoleic and oleic acids. There are two types of EFAs: omega-3 and omega-6 (omega-9 is necessary yet 'non-essential' because the body can manufacture a modest amount on its own, provided essential EFAs are present). EFAs are found in products such as oily fish, nuts and seeds.

VITAMINS AND MINERALS

Vitamins and minerals make our bodies work properly, and although you get vitamins and minerals

You too can get this six-pack with the right nutrition and fitness programme.

from the foods you eat every day, some foods contain more vitamins and minerals than others.

Vitamins

Vitamins fall into two categories: fat soluble and water soluble.

Fat soluble – vitamins A, D, E and K dissolve in fat and can be stored in your body. Some of these stay for a few days, some for up to six months. Then, when it's time for them to be used, your body utilises them.

Water soluble – vitamin C and the B complex vitamins such as vitamins B6, B12, niacin, riboflavin, thiamin, pantothenic acid, biotin, folic acid and folate acid, all need to dissolve in water before your body can absorb them. Because of this, your body cannot store these vitamins. Any vitamin C or B that your body does not use as it passes through your system is lost as waste. So you need a fresh supply of these vitamins every day.

Minerals

Minerals are necessary for three main reasons:

1. Building strong bones and teeth
2. Controlling our cells and body fluids
3. Turning the food we eat into energy

Whereas vitamins are organic substances (made by plants or animals), minerals are inorganic elements that come from the soil and water, and are absorbed by plants or eaten by animals.

Your body needs larger amounts of some minerals, such as calcium, to grow and stay healthy. Other minerals like chromium, copper, iodine, iron, selenium and zinc are called trace minerals, because you only need very small amounts of them each day.

SALT (SODIUM)

Most of our dietary salt comes from the foods we eat, and other salt comes from the drinks we consume.

Both sodium and chloride are essential not only to life, but to good health – it has always been that way. The body's salt/water ratio is critical to a healthy metabolism. The human blood contains 0.9 per cent salt (sodium chloride), and salt maintains the electrolyte balance inside and outside its cells.

Salts are found naturally in food and drink, as well as coming in the form of sea salt, table salt, rock salt etc. There is a good side and a bad side to salt.

The bad side of salt – unnatural/processed salt has been stripped of all the goodness that sea salt provides, such as minerals. Salt makes your body hold on to water, and the extra water stored in your body raises your blood pressure. So the more salt you eat, the higher your blood pressure. The higher your blood pressure, the greater the risk and strain on your heart, arteries, kidneys and brain. This can lead to heart attacks, strokes, dementia and kidney disease.

The good side of salt – sea salt is actually good for you when it is natural and has not been refined. It comes directly from the sea, and not only is it full of minerals, but it can also enhance flavours to make our food taste even better.

Salt is essential to our health and development. We need the vital electrolytes in salt (sodium and potassium) to control water levels in the blood and tissue.

A healthy intake of sea salt aids in balancing:

- Blood sugar levels
- The absorption of food in the intestines
- Acts as a strong and natural anti-histamine
- Can help clear mucus and phlegm from the lungs

We chose not to add any extra salt to any of the recipes in this book, and will leave it up to you whether you add salt to your food for that extra bit of taste. If you do choose to use salt for seasoning, please use sea salt.

HERBS AND SPICES

Herbs and spices add flavour and nutrients to dishes without fat or calories, and are derived from the roots, buds, bark, leaves and fruit of plants.

Herbs are usually the leaves of certain plants, and have been used to treat diseases for thousands of years. Herbs such as basil, chilli, oregano, fenugreek and rosemary are very beneficial to our health.

Many spices contain antioxidants that protect against cancer and heart disease, and can even help with controlling blood sugar. There are other spices with properties that fight E.coli, listeria, *Staphylococcus* and fungus. This is why most of the meals within the 12-week programme have herbs and spices in them.

THE NITTY GRITTY

Rest assured, the nutrition programme is very easy to follow. Whether you are going to commit to the 12-week programme, or if you just want to try the recipes, they are all simple and straightforward to follow. The recipes are not fixed, and you are free to swap the meals around. Even pick a different week entirely if you wish – the choice is yours.

FOLLOWING THE PROGRAMME

The recipes are very easy to follow, and are presented as simple step-by-step instructions. All recipes are designed to feed four people, so remember to halve all quantities if cooking for two or divide by four if it's just for yourself. You will find advice about when to cook tomorrow's lunch, and when you should prepare a marinade for your evening meal. There is a diary for you to fill out too, so you can monitor your own progress.

On each day you will find an easy-to-understand nutritional diary. I used this every day to show exactly what I ate and how I managed to reach her end result. There is a diary for you to fill out too, so you can monitor your own progress.

CHOOSING THE FOODS FOR YOU

When looking through the recipes you may wonder what to do if you don't like one of the key ingredients, such as sweet potato or fish.

The recipes have been designed to be versatile, so that you can swap and change the ingredients to suit you and your taste buds.

Major ingredient alternatives

- Specified fruit → any fruit, not too many grapes though
- Sweet potato → potato, yam, butternut squash
- Baked potato → sweet potato, yam, butternut squash
- Fish → white meat
- Pork → beef
- Chicken → turkey

Choice of foods

When following the 12-week nutritional programme, I would always choose turkey over chicken. Also, to be honest, I didn't consume much skimmed milk (once every two weeks in my muesli). I always chose rice milk/soya milk over skimmed milk.

For the following ingredients I would recommend that you use the same, as they are more beneficial for the body:

- Cold-pressed extra virgin olive oil
- Organic rice milk, unsweetened soya milk and skimmed milk
- Low fat bio live yoghurt
- Organic balsamic vinegar
- Natural organic, or nut and seed, muesli
- Make all of your own sauces and dressings
- Brown sugar
- Free range organic eggs
- Free range poultry and meat from the local butchers
- Fruit juices

The main point to remember when choosing a fruit juice drink is to buy one that is not made from concentrate and is 100 per cent natural, with no added sweeteners or preservatives.

BAD DAY? BAD WEEK? DON'T PANIC!

This is not an eating plan that denies you any naughty foods or treats. I still had the odd off-day. When you do get a bad day, sit back for a moment, analyse what you are doing, and ask yourself:

- Are you eating for the sake of eating?
- Are you eating because you're hungry?
- Have your treat foods got out of hand?
- Are you depriving yourself from snacks/treats?
- Are you missing meals?
- Are you drinking enough water?
- Are you eating or drinking more sugary foods than normal?

Just ask why you are having your bad day, and perhaps you will stop and think before you reach for the bad food.

If you do have a bad day – or an entire bad week – try not to panic. Limit these days as much as possible, but remember this: don't give up. If you hang in there and turn your food back around to being good, you can actually lose more weight than you put on with unhealthy eating. Your body will get a shock, but it will always adapt to its current circumstances.

EATING OUT

Don't panic if you're going to eat out. Look at it as a treat that you deserve from time to time, but of course that doesn't mean run wild and eat what you want. On average I ate out once every three weeks, and all you need to remember is the basics of food.

Perhaps lean towards fish or protein dishes with fresh food, less sauce, and not so many starchy carbohydrates. Foods to avoid when eating out are as follows:

- Creamy dishes
- Starchy carbohydrates
- Deep fried food
- Pan fried food
- Battered food
- Bread
- Chips
- Desserts

Don't be afraid to state how you want your food cooked when ordering. For instance, you may ask for a jacket potato instead of chips, or dressing on the side rather than over your meal. If you do need something sweet after dinner go for fresh fruit, or if you find that too boring share a dessert with someone.

I also recommend that you try to stay clear of take-aways and convenience foods if you can.

TREAT FOODS

You will notice that from time to time I would have foods that would be classed as bad foods or 'treat foods'.

Think of it this way: you are not a robot, and you are not on a diet – you are on a healthy eating plan. This 12-week nutrition programme consists of 80–90 per cent healthy eating, with the rest being considered naughty.

The treat days will also act as motivation, and help keep you on track towards your potential end goal. If, however, you are the sort of person who cannot just have a little treat (you have to finish the entire tub of ice cream), then resist and don't have any treats at all. You know your body – just don't starve it of the nutrients it needs.

I suggest that you don't buy treats on your main shopping trips, and don't leave them out on display. You won't be so tempted to eat them if they're sitting in the cupboard.

DESSERTS AND SNACKS

During the 12-week programme I had two healthy desserts a week, which would normally be yoghurt and fruit, fruit salad with seeds, or just a fruit salad. However, for the first two weeks of the programme I had no desserts at all, and kept to the recipes exactly.

Snacks are just that: snacks. They are not mini meals, so don't treat them as such. Don't purchase snacks that are high in sugar or fat (carbohydrate sugar over 5g or saturated fat over 5g). Surprisingly, this discounts all of the cereal bars on offer at your local supermarket. Try to stay clear of them, as these bars will tend you to give you a sugar craving, which in turn makes you hungry.

Listed below is a suggested list of snacks you could eat. The quantities listed are what I had on average each week.

Snack list

- Melon, mango or coconut – 1 to share
- Peach, plum, or kiwi – 1
- Pineapple – 1 to share
- Orange or nectarine – 1
- Berries (blackberries, goji, blueberries, raspberries or strawberries) – 2 portions
- Pear – 1
- Banana – 5
- Apple – 5
- Wholegrain crispbread – 3
- Crackers/flat breads – 1
- Small bowl of muesli (if really hungry) – 2
- Yoghurt/soya yoghurt (four dessert spoons) – 1
- Nuts (cashew, pine or occasionally mixed nuts) – 2 to 3 handfuls
- Soya nuts – 3 to 4 handfuls after training sessions
- Seeds (pumpkin or sunflower) – 2 to 3 handfuls
- Pitta bread/wrap with salad and protein filling – 1

Roughly speaking, I would snack four to five times a day at random intervals. You can use this as a guide, but you don't have to snack five times a day – just when you need to.

CAFFEINE AND ALCOHOL

As part of the 12-week fitness and nutritional programme, I chose to live a healthy lifestyle that did not cut out any essential dietary needs, but also not to completely remove the sociable side of my lifestyle, which included drinking alcohol, tea and coffee. I simply chose the healthier option when doing so. For example, when I had a choice between teas or coffees, I chose green tea, herbal tea, or decaffeinated tea and coffee. When I was drinking alcohol, I avoided beer and opted for a spirit like vodka with a fruit or diet mixer.

During the 12-week programme you may have parties to go to, or you might meet up with friends at your local pub. Here is a little advice as to what to choose:

- Spirit with fruit or diet mixer over ales/lager/beer
- Red wine over white wine
- Guinness or ale over beer/lager
- Cider over beer/lager

On average I consumed a little over one alcoholic drink per week. The average alcohol unit consumption was 2.4 per week, which is the equivalent of having one pint of beer or two single spirits with a diet mixer a week.

RELISHES AND DRESSINGS

Here are some great healthy dressings that you can make easily at home and are used in the weekly recipes:

Houmous

1 large can chickpeas, drained
2 cloves garlic
2–3 tablespoons olive oil
1 dessertspoon tahini (sesame seed spread)

Tzatziki

1 clove garlic, crushed
200g yoghurt
¼ cucumber, finely grated
½ red onion, finely chopped
1 tablespoon parsley, chopped
1 tablespoon mint, chopped

Avocado relish

2 avocados, peeled and chopped
1 tablespoon lime juice
½ small red onion, finely cut
2 tomatoes, chopped

Relish

1 bunch fresh parsley
6 anchovy fillets
Zest of 2 lemons, grated
115ml lemon juice
60ml olive oil

Mint dressing

150g yoghurt
2 tablespoons mint, chopped
½ tablespoon olive oil
2 tablespoons lemon juice

Basil dressing

1 tablespoon olive oil

1 clove garlic, crushed
1 tablespoon lemon juice
1 tablespoon basil leaves, shredded

Salad dressing
4 tablespoons yoghurt
¼ cucumber, grated
1 tablespoon olive oil
1 tablespoon balsamic vinegar
2 teaspoons black pepper
2 teaspoons dried dill

Nutty delight dressing
3 tablespoons olive oil
3 tablespoons yoghurt
Sprinkle of pine nuts
½ tablespoon balsamic vinegar
Black pepper

Mustard dressing
1 tablespoon Dijon mustard
1 tablespoon olive oil
2 teaspoons cider vinegar
1 teaspoon water

Dill dressing
1 tablespoon fresh dill, chopped
250g yoghurt
1 clove garlic, crushed
1 teaspoon balsamic vinegar

All-purpose dressing
2 tablespoon olive oil
1 tablespoon balsamic vinegar
1 clove garlic, crushed
1 teaspoon dijon mustard
Black pepper

Ginger dressing for the wok
2 tablespoons light soy sauce
2 teaspoons lime juice
1 teaspoon ginger, grated

Spicy dressing 1
2 tablespoons lime juice
1 tablespoon fish sauce

1 tablespoon light soy sauce
1 clove garlic, crushed
1 red chilli, de-seeded and chopped

Spicy dressing 2
1 red chilli, finely sliced
½ teaspoon ground cumin
1 tablespoon lime juice

Coriander and yoghurt dressing
500g yoghurt
2 tablespoons coriander, chopped
1 clove garlic, finely chopped
4 teaspoons lemon juice
1 teaspoon ground cumin

FOOD PORTIONS AND PRESENTATION
Within each recipe and shopping list, all the ingredients that you will need for breakfast, lunch and dinner are listed. This is just a guideline, as sometimes (for example, during the week) you might eat two turkey breasts instead of the one recommended, or increase the muesli recommended for breakfast to give you the energy you need for the day ahead. Bear in mind that all recipes are designed for four people, so adjust quantities according to how many people you are cooking for.

Surprisingly, the presentation of your food is almost as important as how it tastes. It has been proven that good food presentation can make your food taste better due to your brain perceiving that the food looks delicious and smells delectable before even tasting it. So take your time with all your meal presentations.

SHOPPING LISTS
Items in the shopping lists are organised in alphabetical order under categories of fish, meat, dairy, carbohydrates, fruit, vegetables, herbs and spices, and other. This will help you be in and out of the supermarket with more ease and efficiency. All the lists have been designed to cover every meal, but you do need to add healthy snacks to your list.

When you start, you will notice that the amounts are very precise, but these are just recommendations. For instance, if you cannot find 12 tomatoes, only a pack of eight, don't worry because the recipes are adaptable.

If, for example, you don't like to eat sweet potatoes or butternut squash, you can eat yam instead. If you would rather eat turkey instead of chicken because it is leaner and healthier, you can. You are the boss, just be good to yourself.

It is important when you are shopping to not worry so much about the calories, but look carefully at the carbohydrates (sugars), and the fats (saturated) that you are popping into your supermarket trolley.

SHOPPING LIST **WEEK 1**		
CARBOHYDRATES 1 bag of brown rice 480g of muesli 1 bag of pine nuts 8 wholemeal/brown pitta breads 240g porridge oats 4 jacket potatoes 1 bag of sunflower seeds 1 bag of pumpkin seeds 9 sweet potatoes 4 organic tortilla wraps Wheat biscuits **DAIRY AND NON-DAIRY ALTERNATIVES** 350g low fat cottage cheese/ soft goat's cheese 8 eggs 40g feta/goat's cheese 1 light soft cheese/soft goat's cheese 680ml skimmed/ soya/rice/ oat milk 2kg soya/plain yoghurt **FISH** 8 anchovy fillets 4 mackerel fillets 4 salmon fillets 1 pack of smoked salmon 4 small tuna cans 350g tuna steaks **MEAT** 4 200g beef steaks 8 chicken breasts 400g lean ham 8 turkey breasts 1.4kg rack of veal	**FRUIT** 6 apples 12 bananas 1 punnet of blueberries 2 lemons 2 mangos 1 orange 1 large pineapple 1 punnet of raspberries **VEGETABLES** 1 avocado 2 bags of baby spinach 25g black olives 3 butternut squash 5 carrots 2 celery sticks 2 courgettes 1 cucumber 175g French beans 2 leeks 4 lettuces 265g mangetout 150g mushrooms 1 onion 115g plum tomatoes 5 red onions 5 red peppers 20 red tomatoes 100g rocket salad 26 spring onions 1 bag of sweet corn 2 yellow peppers **HERBS** Basil Black pepper Chinese five-spice Coriander Cumin	Dill Fresh ginger 1 garlic bulb Green chilli Ground coriander Mint Nutmeg Paprika Turmeric **OTHER** Balsamic vinegar Beef stock Corn flour Chicken stock Cold-pressed extra virgin olive oil Ginger wine Soy sauce Tandoori paste Tomato purée **SNACKS** Fruit Wholegrain crispbread/ crackers/flat breads Small bowl of muesli Soya yoghurt Nuts (cashew, pine or occasionally mixed nuts) Soya nuts Seeds (pumpkin or sunflower) **FRUIT DRINKS** 1 carton fruit juice drink

WHEN TO EAT

There is a lot of stipulation on what time you should eat. We all have different lifestyles and routines, but sometimes it is just physically impossible to eat at a certain time. All you have to remember is that you need to eat breakfast, lunch and dinner – do not worry too much about the timings. If you are eating later in the day keep your food portions smaller than normal, increase the protein and decrease your carbohydrate intake.

WHEN TO EAT ON TRAINING DAYS

The food we eat before and after exercise is important both for comfort and for performance.

The major source of fuel for active muscles is carbohydrate, which is stored in the muscles as glycogen. It takes time to fill glycogen stores completely, and what you eat following exercise either helps or hinders this process.

You should aim to eat 1.5 hours before or after exercise. Again, in reality this is just a rough timing to help as a guide. Sometimes you might eat breakfast and be cycling to work within 40 minutes, so just listen to your body and decide what's right for you. When you finish exercise, try to eat protein within 30 minutes to fuel your muscles and help them repair. I use soya nuts as my post-exercise snack.

FOODS THAT NORMALLY HELPS WITH PERFORMANCE BEFORE EXERCISE

As glucose is the preferred energy source for most exercises, the meal before should contain carbohydrates that are easy to digest, plus protein and a small amount fat. For example, a turkey salad wrap or soya nuts with a piece of fruit or a fruit smoothie.

FOODS TO AVOID BEFORE EXERCISE

Foods that are high in fat and/or fibre are digested slowly and remain in the stomach longer, so try to avoid these. These foods include meat, chips, chocolate bars and cakes.

EXERCISING ON A FULL STOMACH

This is not ideal, as any food remaining on your stomach can cause cramp, stitches, nausea or even diarrhoea. To make sure you have enough energy while exercising you should eat between one and four hours beforehand, depending on the type and quantity of food you are eating. Remember, everyone's different so we recommend experimenting to find out what works best for you.

EXERCISING IN THE MORNING

If you are the sort of person who exercises early in the morning, or you have a big race that day, then it's best to wake up a little bit early to ensure you have your pre-exercise meal (breakfast) and enough energy to perform to the best of your ability. The closer you are to performing your exercise, the less you should be eating.

EXERCISING IN THE EVENING

You can either choose to train before or after your evening meal. It is completely up to you. If you prefer to train straight after work, ensure you eat a healthy snack at least one hour before you exercise, and then eat within an hour – or preferably half an hour – of finishing.

However, if you choose to train after dinner, take into account what we've already mentioned about exercising on a full stomach – work out what is going to be best for you.

The most important thing to remember is to hydrate before and after exercise.

WHAT YOU EAT AFTER EXERCISE

The first thing to do after any exercise is to drink water, replacing any fluids you will have lost.

It is then very important that you replace your glycogen stores and consume carbohydrates (such as a piece of fruit) within 15 minutes. The reason for this is that carbohydrate consumption stimulates insulin production, which aids muscle glycogen production (repairing your body faster).

If within half an hour you can also consume protein with the carbohydrates, the insulin response almost doubles. The protein provides the amino acids necessary to rebuild muscle tissue that will have been damaged during training.

In short, to give your body the best possible chance of recovery and repair after strenuous exercise you should aim to eat a 4 to 1 ratio of carbohydrate and protein within half an hour of finishing.

FREQUENTLY ASKED QUESTIONS

WILL I GET BORED WITH THE 12-WEEK NUTRITION PLAN?

The recipes have been created so that you don't eat the same meals each week and you have a different dinner recipe every day for the whole 12 weeks. With this wide variety and varied cooking, your taste buds should not be feeling neglected.

WILL I BE ABLE TO FEED THE WHOLE FAMILY?

This is a plan based around a family of four.

WILL I GET HUNGRY?

To be honest, there will be times when you will feel hungrier than usual, but there will also be days where you feel full. When you first start the programme your body and eating habits will change, so you will probably find that the first two weeks are the most demanding. The programme has been particularly devised to fulfil your appetite with tantalising meals that will keep hunger at bay.

On some days of the fitness programme you may require more food for certain days. Follow the plan and use my diary as a guide, and you should end up getting where you want to be.

ARE THE SHOPPING LISTS EASY TO FOLLOW?

Items on the shopping lists have been organised according to common categories, as well as being in alphabetical order. This will enable you to shop quickly and easily. You can access them online and print them off to take to the supermarket.

DID YOU USE SUPPLEMENTS?

No. This is mainly to show that if you are on the right healthy eating plan, then you don't need any supplements. Having said that, I am not against supplements as some of them are beneficial for the body.

TRAINING BASICS AND SET-UP

04

The 12-week programme will be very challenging, both mentally and physically. It will change your fitness levels, physical shape, confidence, posture, skin and eating habits – and hopefully change you into what you want to become.

This chapter looks at the basics of weight training, running and cycling, and then the set-up and equipment needed to complete the programme.

WEIGHT TRAINING
REPETITIONS (REPS)

A rep is a contraction of the muscle followed by the extension – for example, arm-curling the dumbbell up and back down to the start.

The general rule:

- Upper body: 6–10 reps
- Lower body: 12–16 reps
- Strength training: 1–6 reps

- For size: 6–12 reps
- Muscular endurance: 15+ reps

When you start your reps you should be pushing about 70–80 per cent of your maximum effort, and by the end of the last set you should be at 80–100 per cent of your maximum effort.

SETS

A set is a specific number of repetitions performed for different exercises.

The general rule is, the larger the muscle groups (e.g. thighs, back and chest), the more sets. Normally you would aim for around 12 sets per large muscle group, while bodybuilders go up to 20 sets or more if required. For smaller muscle groups (e.g. biceps and triceps) you need to do fewer sets, usually around 9–12 sets. These are just average recommendations.

FULL RANGE OF MOTION

Full range of motion enables the entire muscle to be contracted by up to 90–100 per cent, instead of, say, only 50 per cent with a partial rep. There are some exceptions if you are doing specific advanced training that involves partial or half reps.

When I performed my exercises, it was important to note how many repetitions and sets per exercise I completed, plus the technique and full range of motion.

TECHNIQUE

Technique is the most fundamental part of training. When you perform with a good technique you ensure maximum muscle contraction and minimum injury to your muscles.

It is important to choose the appropriate weight for the exercise to maintain quality of technique. If you are trying to isolate a muscle group and you're lifting too heavy a weight, your technique will be altered, so that other muscles will become involved in helping you perform that exercise.

Remember – it is the quality of the movement, and not quantity.

RESTING BETWEEN SETS

Choosing how much time you spend resting between your sets depends on how you are training. Either way, you do not want your muscles to recover too much, but just enough to continue your workout, unless you are after strength training.

I tended to rest between one and three minutes on the weight training sessions. During circuits and endurance-type exercises, I didn't rest at all between any sets. This is to keep both the heart rate up and the muscles full of blood and lactic acid.

BREATHING

When people are training, they seem always to worry about how they breathe when lifting weights. The general rule when breathing should be:

- Exhale on the way out for effort.
- Inhale after effort.

For example, while bench pressing exhale when pushing the bar up and inhale as the bar comes down to your chest.

RATING PERCEIVED EXERTION (RPE)

This scale is handy to describe the intensity of training sessions. I have used the RPE throughout my training sessions to show you how hard I trained. Use the same scale for your own training to monitor your progress:

0 Nothing at all
1 Very, very light
2 Very light
3 Fairly light
4 Light
5 Moderate
6 Fairly hard
7 Hard
8 Very hard
9 Very, very hard
10 Maximum effort possible

The RPE in cardiovascular (CV) sessions shows you the intensity of how hard and fast to run. For instance, if it was 7/10 for running, that would convert to running at 70 per cent effort. You will see I ran most of the short distances at 90 per cent.

TRAINING AVERAGE RPE

7/10 = 70 per cent of rate of exertion per training session.

ENERGY AVERAGE RPE

You can apply the RPE scale to anything, such as

This is me on day 1, week 1 – you can see me focusing on the technique.

your energy levels: 0 = not much energy at all and 10 = maximum energy.

STRESS AVERAGE RPE

In the training diary the RPE scale is used for recording stress: 0 = not much stress at all and 10 = maximum stress.

GYM SET-UP

I was lucky enough to be able to set up a gym in my own garage. I know most people have gym memberships now, but if you are not able to access a fully equipped gym, I recommend the purchase of dumbbells and a bench. You will need somewhere to do pull-ups and a floor mat for the floor exercises.

EQUIPMENT

The equipment listed below should give you everything you require.

Weights

(You don't need to buy both adjustable weights, just buy the appropriate ones for you.)

- Adjustable dumbbells 5lbs (2.25kg) to 52.5lbs (24kg)
- Adjustable dumbbells 10lbs (4.5kg) to 90lbs (41kg)
- 150kg Olympic weights and 7 foot Olympic bar
- Bench
- Rack and cable

Attachments
- Single handle
- Rope
- Lat pull-down bar with rack and cable bar
- Close grip handle
- If required, Olympic adjustment, from standard size bar diameter to Olympic size diameter

Other
- Bosu
- 4kg or 8kg kettle bell
- Abs mat
- Step box
- Full-length mirror (for correcting your technique)

RUNNING
TECHNIQUE
The type of surface will determine how you run. For example, when running on soft surfaces like sand you should run in other people's tracks or by shuffling and digging your toes into the sand. This will use your calves more than when running on hard surfaces.

When running on hard surfaces, the general rule is a heel to toe contact. As your heel comes into contact with the ground it rolls along the foot and you then push off using the toes. Keeping your stride open keeps the stress off your knees and hips and sends it through your body.

You need to relax your whole upper body to enable your heart, lungs and legs to work more effectively. If you run with your hands clenched, for instance, blood will be taken from your legs and other areas needed for running and be put into your clenched hands. In turn, this results in decreasing your effectiveness in running. Your arms should be relaxed and in rhythm with your feet.

BREATHING
The most important part of running is finding your rhythm, whether this is from breathing or by your strides. Either way, this enables you to relax so that your breathing becomes deeper in inhalation and exhalation. What we are trying to prevent here is shortness of breath. This results in oxygen being deprived from your muscles, which can cause cramp.

RUNNING SET-UP
GAIT
It is very important to wear the correct footwear when training, and especially when running. You can go to a specialist running shop, where they will look at your feet and running style and prescribe trainers especially for you. Or, you can do a simple home test and prescribe your own trainers. Once you know your feet, it is easier for you to look for a pair of trainers to suit you. You need to look to see if you pronate, supinate, or neither.

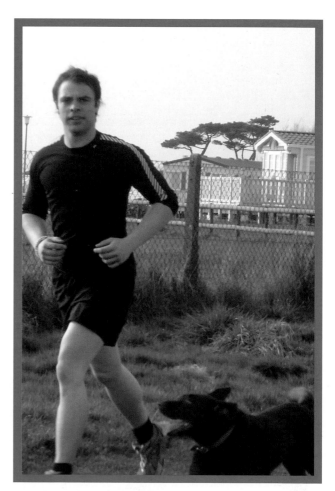

Here I am running with my dog right at the start of my 12-week programme.

Knowing your foot type – home test

To establish your foot type at home, the quickest way is to wet your feet and then stand on a dry area, so you can clearly see an imprint of your feet.

From the pictures below you can determine what foot type you have.

Supinated foot – high arch: foot doesn't roll over before toe-off, foot strike

Over-pronated foot – flat foot: foot rolls in excessively during foot strike but rolls to the inside

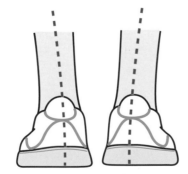

Neutral foot: ideal biomechanics

TRAINERS

What to look for in trainers: comfort, durability, performance, weight, style and price.

Types of trainers:

- Neutral/cushioning – neutral biomechanics
- Anti-pronation – over-pronators
- Motion control – biomechanical disorders and pronation control
- Racers – light, neutral and flexible

CLOTHING

- Running socks
- Cycling shorts
- Running shorts
- Breathable sports top
- Trainers
- Speed and distance watch

CYCLING

TECHNIQUE

After setting up the bike, the correct cycling technique will require you to push through the ball of your foot on the way down while pulling the pedal up with your hip flexors – push and pull. When attempting a hill, you will need either to shuffle back on the seat to push and pull with more power, or to stand.

Comfort and efficiency in cycling must go hand in hand. You need to find a relaxed and comfortable position. You should never sacrifice comfort for speed. You need to concentrate on maintaining a still upper body – by relaxing your shoulders you can help conserve your energy.

BREATHING

You need to find your own rhythm, which will enable you to relax into your cycle.

CADENCE

Learning to cycle at a high cadence is going to be the best fundamental skill you can learn. You should be aiming for a cadence between 80rpm and 90rpm, or if you're strong in cycling try to reach 100rpm.

To count your cadence all you need to do is count the number of revolutions you pedal over 15 seconds, then multiply it by four.

BIKE SET-UP

Type of bike

I spent a year cycling to and from work, and I know that it is important to get the best bike to suit your pocket, but also one that suits your cycling needs, depending on the type of cycling you do.

The type of bike you require depends on the type of surface you will be cycling on and what you want to use it for. Use the list below to understand what factors you need to consider:

- Type – off-road, road or hybrid
- Performance
- Maintenance
- Weight
- Comfort
- Style

The bike I used was a hybrid tri-cross. I chose this bike because it best suits the conditions for me.

Bike frame – to get the correct frame size for you should go to a specialist bike shop and allow them to fit you out with the correct size.

Saddle height – prop yourself up against a wall or get a friend to hold your bike. Place one heel on the pedal at the lowest point of the revolution – that leg should be straight but not locked out. This incorporates the use of the quadriceps muscles.

Saddle position – at 3 o'clock, the anterior aspect of the patella (front of the kneecap) should line up

with the centre of the pedal axle. To achieve this you can move the saddle forwards or backwards, as well as tilting the saddle up and down.

Tyre pressure – for a road bike with 700c high-pressure wheels, the correct pressure will be around 100 to 120psi. For a mountain bike being ridden off-road the tyre pressure will be anywhere from 35 to 60psi.

The psi varies with each manufacturer, so please check the recommendations on the sidewall of the tyre first.

CYCLING EQUIPMENT

Clothing
- Windproof T-shirt
- Windproof jacket
- Lightweight waterproof jacket
- Cycling gloves
- Cycling shorts
- Cycling shoes

Other
- Bike bag
- Waterproof dry bag
- Water bottle/hydration pack
- Speed and distance bike computer
- Pedals with/without clips
- Pump
- Bell
- Adjustable allen keys
- Spare inner tube
- Puncture repair kit
- First-aid kit

WHEN TO TRAIN

You can train at any time throughout the 12-week programme. You just have to choose what time suits you to get the most out of your workouts, whether it is first thing in the morning or last thing at night.

REST AND RECOVERY

Rest days are almost as important as training days. It's during sleep and rest that your body recuperates from all its hard work, repairing and building your muscles to become more toned, stronger and fitter. You should have total rest on the specified rest days.

Our bodies don't respond well to extremes. For example, if you eat too much you gain weight. However, if you eat too few calories, your body shuts down and your weight loss screeches to a halt. The same goes for exercise. You need to find a happy medium to coax your body to change in the way you want it to.

WHY SHOULD YOU REST AND RECOVER AFTER TRAINING?

Your body doesn't become stronger when you work out, but when you rest. For example, when you lift weights, you create little tears within your muscle fibres (which is good, so don't worry). When you rest, the muscle fibres begin to repair themselves, growing back stronger than before. So, as your muscles grow and become stronger, you are able to lift more weight. If you don't allow those muscles adequate rest, however, the fibres won't have a chance to heal, and may even weaken, until eventually you could even injure yourself with a pull or a tear.

Recovery is influenced by many factors, including healthy eating, hydration and sleep. There are also more complex factors such as work and family stress. You need to be aware of the influence your personal lifestyle can have on your recovery.

If it is clear you are not overtraining, then consider if your lifestyle could be the cause of your deterioration. If you are experiencing stress at work or at home, try reducing the number, duration and intensity of your training sessions. Below are some tips on how to achieve this.

Active rest – you can help flush out lactic acid and other waste products that build in your muscles by doing very gentle exercise, such as walking or a very light swim or cycle. The key is to enjoy the activity and not to work your muscles too hard.

Passive rest – do no activities at all. Enjoy a day off seeing family or friends, or just lazing around at home. The choice is yours.

Stretching – stretching can help increase the range of movement and efficiency of muscles, reduce the likelihood and seriousness of injury, extend your training life, and reduce muscle fatigue and soreness. Stretching can easily be incorporated into your day – for example, when at your desk, or even while watching television.

Spa benefits – soak in a spa or use the sauna to help your muscles recover faster. You can try to stretch while in the spa. Alternating hot and cold water in the shower helps flush out waste products and bring oxygen to tired muscles.

Refuel – the body is most efficient at absorbing nutrients straight after training. Eating immediately after your workout supports the body's need to repair itself.

Sleep – it is during sleep that the growth hormone sets to work, protein production occurs, and our mind and body are recharged. The amount of sleep required varies from person to person, but most people fully recover after between seven and nine hours sleep.

Rehydrate – the harder you train, the more water you need to drink. Drinking enough before and immediately after your workout is your key to success.

FITNESS TESTS

You should take fitness tests at the start of your training programme, and every four weeks, to monitor your progress and your eventual results. Ongoing testing acts as a morale booster, and highlights areas in which you are not performing to the best of your abilities. By taking the following fitness tests every four weeks, it gives your body the time and opportunity to adapt and get fitter and stronger.

BLEEP TEST

The bleep test measures your aerobic fitness level over a 20-metre distance. It involves you running continuously between two lines measured 20 metres apart, in time with the audio bleeps.

Scoring on the bleep test

Use the table overleaf to assess your individual scores taken during the bleep test.

Level	Speed (km/h)	Shuttles	Distance (m)	Cumulative distance (m)
1	8.5	8	160	160
2	9.0	8	160	320
3	9.5	8	160	480
4	10.0	9	180	660
5	10.5	9	180	840
6	11.0	10	200	1040
7	11.5	10	200	1240
8	12.0	10	200	1440
9	12.5	11	220	1660
10	13.0	11	220	1880
11	13.5	12	240	2120
12	14.0	12	240	2360
13	14.5	13	260	2620
14	15.0	13	260	2880
15	15.5	13	260	3140
16	16.0	14	280	3420
17	16.5	14	280	3700
18	17.0	15	300	4000
19	17.5	15	300	4300
20	18.0	15	300	4600
21	18.5	16	320	4920
22	19.0	16	320	5240
23	19.5	17	340	5580

You will start off with a slow speed, which will gradually increase as the levels increase. At the end of each level you will hear the bleeps getting closer together, which continues each minute.

If you have reached the line before the bleep, you must wait until you hear the bleep before running again.

Note: if the line is not reached in time with the bleep you have a chance to turn and catch up the pace for two more bleeps. The test is stopped if you are unable to reach the line in two consecutive ends, or if you fail to reach the line with a 2m gap.

Bleep test equipment
• Tape measure to measure the distance
• Cones or some type of markers
• Bleep test audio track

The bleep test audio track is commercially available at very low cost (or even free) as a CD or as a download to play on laptop, iPad, etc. Enter 'bleep test' in a search engine to find the many options.

Results for bleep test
The results below are not predictions for maximal oxygen uptake, but are indicators for aerobic fitness. Each score shows the test level and the number of shuttles completed successfully (e.g. 4/6 = level 4 and 6 shuttles completed).

Age	Excellent	Good	Average	Fair	Poor
14–16	10/9	9/1	6/7	5/1	4/7
17–20	10/11	9/3	6/8	5/2	4/9
21–30	10/8	9/2	6/6	5/1	4/9
31–41	10/4	8/7	6/3	4/6	4/5
41–50	9/9	7/2	5/7	4/2	4/1

MUSCULAR ENDURANCE TESTS

In the following tests you have one minute to perform as many repetitions as you can. This will be a good guide to your muscular endurance, as well as being a great way of motivating yourself to do better.

The results shown are from my years in the fitness industry, and represent an average of what I have recorded and seen. See Chapter 7 for guidance on how to perform these exercises.

Press-ups

Do full press-ups if you can, otherwise ¾ press-ups.

Age	17–19	20–29	30–39	40–49	50–59	60–65
Excellent	>56	>47	>41	>34	>31	>30
Good	47–55	39–46	34–40	28–33	25–30	24–29
Above average	35–46	30–39	25–33	21–27	18–24	17–23
Average	19–34	17–29	13–24	11–20	9–17	6–16
Below average	11–18	10–16	8–12	6–10	5–8	3–5
Poor	4–10	4–9	2–7	1–5	1–4	1–2
Very poor	<4	<4	<2	0	0	0

Squats

Do full squats to test your leg endurance.

Age	18–25	26–35	36–45	46–55	56–65	65+
Excellent	>49	>45	>41	>35	>31	>28
Good	44–48	40–44	35–40	29–34	25–30	22–27
Above average	39–43	35–39	30–34	25–38	21–24	19–21
Average	35–38	31–34	27–29	22–24	17–20	15–18
Below average	31–34	29–30	23–26	18–21	13–16	11–14
Poor	25–30	22–28	17–22	13–17	9–12	7–10
Very poor	<25	<22	<17	<9	<9	<7

Half sit-ups

To test your abdominal endurance, half sit-ups and not full ones.

Age	Under 35	35–45	Over 45
Excellent	60	50	40
Good	45	40	25
Average	30	25	15
Below average	15	10	5

Dips

Completed as a bench dip. The average I have seen with dips for men is between 45 and 60.

Excellent	75+
Good	55 – 74
Average	35 – 54
Below average	35 and under

Pull-ups

There is no time limit, but you must keep hanging from your hands and keep your feet off the floor at all times.

The average result for pull-ups I have seen for men is 6–10. The best I have ever seen was 51 by a Royal Marine.

1 rep max

One repetition maximum (1RM) is the maximum amount of weight one can lift in a single repetition for a given exercise.

When performing 1RM, make sure you have warmed up properly. Perform 3–4 sets before attempting 1RM. You should always have a training partner with you for your safety.

I would perform a 1RM every four weeks to test the muscle's total strength. The following exercises are compound movements that test more than one muscle group:

- Bench press
- Military press
- Squats
- Deadlifts

LET'S GET STARTED

05

Within the 12-week fitness programme you will go through over 60 different workouts and use over 80 different exercises to get the body you want to achieve. We will look at the basic training methods, warm-ups, cool-downs and quick stretches to get the most out of your muscles.

WEIGHT TRAINING

I am sure you have seen those people who use the gym regularly but have bodies that never change shape. This is due to several different reasons, but the main ones are:

- Lack of knowledge and technique
- No variety – using the same routine continuously
- Never increasing their performance (e.g. not increasing the weights when lifting)

We need to use as many different methods while training to get the most out of our bodies. This will encourage our bodies to get bigger and stronger, as our bodies won't become accustomed to the same routine.

Have a look through the different types of training methods I used, and take note so that you can use it to do your best.

SUPERSETS

These are two exercises performed in a row without stopping. For example, perform a bent-over row followed by pec fly.

Static lunges (bosu)	Superset sets and reps	Squat thrusts
3 × 15		3 × 15

For example, this superset means completing 3 sets of 15 reps of static lunges and 3 sets of 15 reps of squats. Perform the first of three sets of static lunges, followed by the first set of three squats without stopping. After performing the first set of both exercises you can rest, then repeat until you have completed three sets of both exercises.

DROP SETS

Perform an exercise with a heavy weight to reach failure (see opposite page). Lower the weight and reach failure again. Keep lowering the weight until specified.

PYRAMID TRAINING

This has a warm-up, a maximum and a cool-down all in one. Begin at the bottom of the left side of the pyramid and climb up until you are all the way at the top and then come back down on the right hand side to the base. The numbers represent the repetitions.

Set 1 = 1 pull-up, set 2 = 2 pull-ups . . . set 10 = 10 pull-ups.

NEGATIVE TRAINING

You can use negative training with weights by getting someone to lift the concentric part of the action, and then you slowly lower the weight, under control, back to the start over a count of five. This feels strange as you are performing it, but by the time you have finished you will have a nice big pump.

CHEATING

When you hit failure within your set you can perform cheat reps. Try to keep good form and, by utilising other muscles/muscle groups to help you, you can

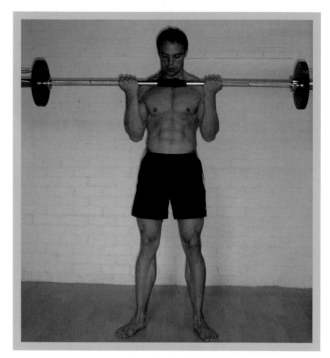

Warming up ready to lift some heavy weights.

lift the weight so that you can still target the muscle that you want. For example, when I was doing arm curls, I was on my final set and only managed to get four repetitions, so I did a cheat by involving my deltoids and back – but not too much to take away the stress placed on my biceps.

NEGATIVE PULL-UPS

Use negative pull-ups if you are unable to perform more than five repetitions in a row. Negative pull-ups will build you up nice and quickly, so eventually you will be able to perform more than 10 reps in a row.

Start with your chin at bar level either by stepping on a step box or object or by getting your training partner to lift you up to the top (with a little help from yourself). Slowly lower yourself over a count of five seconds back down to the bottom, until your arms are straight. This counts as one negative rep. Then repeat the number of reps specified.

PRESS-UPS

With all of the press-ups you will be performing over the next 12 weeks, you must be able to perform at least 30 in a minute. If you are unable to perform 30 regular press-ups, you should be looking to perform ¾ press-ups. As soon as you can perform more than 60 in a row, you should then be able to perform 30 regular press-ups.

If you find you prefer the ¾ press-ups, you can do all of them throughout the 12 weeks like this, but of course you will get more results from doing full press-ups.

FAILURE

To train to failure, you continue a set until you can't do any more repetitions with that weight without stopping or losing technique.

Example:

- 1st set: warm-up set, 20 reps
- 2nd set: add weight that allows your muscles to fail between 10 and 15 reps
- 3rd set: add more weight to allow your muscles to fail between 6 and 10 reps
- 4th set: using the same weight, allow your muscles to fail between 6 and 10 reps

FORCED REP

Get your training partner to spot you, to force extra reps to complete your set.

I used this method with my training partner towards the end of the 12-week programme. I never noted it on the diary, but as a general rule I performed this from week 8 onwards, almost every session.

WEIGHTS

Throughout the book I have noted the total weights in kilos/pounds to show you how much I was lifting. The total includes the weight of the bar.

Please remember that I have trained for most of my life, apart from the five months prior to beginning the 12-week programme, so I was able to lift slightly more than some people when they first go to the gym. Use the programme as a guide, and don't worry about lifting the same weight as me. But if you can lift the same, or you can go heavier, please do so.

CARDIOVASCULAR TRAINING
UPPER BODY PT (PHYSICAL TRAINING)

Throughout the programme the upper body PT are exercises that use no equipment, such as pull-ups, dips, press-ups, etc.

Example of upper body PT

Regular press-ups	× 10
½ sit-ups	× 10
Diamond press-ups	× 10
Leg levers	× 10
Wide press-ups	× 10
Full sit-ups	× 10

All six exercises should be completed in order from the top to the bottom, and all within two minutes. This counts as one cycle. Repeat 19 more cycles in sequence. This should last no more than 40 minutes.

PULL-UP WORKOUT

Regular – 2, 4, 6, 8, 10
Reverse – 2, 4, 6, 8, 10
Close – 2, 4, 6, 8, 10
Wide – 2, 4, 6, 8, 10
Mountain Climber – 2, 4, 6, 8, 10
Start first with regular pull-ups and complete all five sets with no more than 30 seconds to one minute rest in between. Then move on to the reverse pull-ups and complete the next five sets. Repeat until you have completed all five pull-ups in this way. Trust me, when you get to the last few sets you will feel the greatest pump in your back, and you will also feel exhausted.

RUN PT

I enjoy running and exercising outside, so if you can, try to perform the running and exercises outside instead of in a gym.

Run for the specified distance and then perform the exercise with the number of sets and repetitions required, before moving on to the next exercise or run with no rest in between.

The running should be at 75 per cent of your maximum effort (RPE 7.5/10), and the exercises should be with good technique and as fast as you can to keep your heart rate up.

CYCLE PT

This is to be done in the same fashion as the run PT.

This was one of the toughest workouts I completed in the 12-week programme.

RUNNING

Start the running nice and slow, as you want to have a steady build-up phase for your fitness. It is all about getting outside and running.

The short distance running is about timings. After the 3rd week, once you have attained some base fitness, you should time your 3-mile run, and from then on either aim to beat or match your previous/best times.

On the longer runs, I just tried to keep in my aerobic zone most of the way. This should be a comfortable pace, at which you should be able to hold a conversation with your training partner. If, however, you find it hard to talk, you are probably running too hard and you are out of your aerobic zone.

HILL AND STEP TRAINING

Choose a hill that takes no longer than one minute to sprint up to the top. The emphasis is on the word 'sprint', because that is how we keep in our anaerobic zone and get fitter.

With the step training choose a staircase that takes you roughly 30 seconds to sprint up to the top, touching every step on the way up. You can alternatively count the same number of steps that I ran up and do the same.

CYCLING

I recommend you time either a particular route or distance, and each session you complete it again try to match the same time or, if possible, beat it. Of course, you will notice that your time varies depending on the prior training, weather conditions, and how you are feeling that day. If you are down on your time, take these influences into account and try not to worry too much.

CIRCUITS

When exercising in circuit training, the most important thing is to push yourself as hard as you can and never rest in between any exercise or CV-based exercise.

You should try to lift as much as you can, doing as many reps as you can, running as fast as you can, and so on. All of this helps target fat loss, muscle building and heart/lung fitness.

WARM-UP

The warm-up is to prime your muscles, heart and lungs in preparation for your training session. You should slowly increase your intensity as you go through your workout, which will increase your heart rate and blood pressure.

CARDIOVASCULAR (CV) TRAINING SESSIONS

Use five minutes before you start your CV session to perform the same exercise, but gradually build-up the intensity until you feel that your body is thoroughly warmed up.

WEIGHT AND CIRCUIT TRAINING SESSIONS

The following routine warms up all your muscles and systems, and takes about five minutes.

Arm circle forwards and backwards

Start with a small circle forwards about the size of a golf ball and gradually increase the circle size until you are rotating them to the maximum. For the arm circle backwards repeat by going in reverse.

Breast stroke and reverse breast stroke

Perform the breast stroke technique used for swimming. As you are going through the technique make sure you are really stretching forwards, and on the way back try to open up your chest to feel a stretch in your pectorals.

For reverse breast stroke, repeat by going in reverse.

Front crawl and back stroke

The front crawl is the same as the swimming technique. When performing, make sure you're really trying to rotate each arm forwards and allow your hips to move with the movement. Reverse the direction in the same way for the back stroke.

Butterfly stroke forwards and backwards

The butterfly stroke is the same as the swimming technique. As you are performing the stroke gradually increase the speed of the rotations forwards and then backwards.

Military Press

Perform the military press movement, trying to feel a little burn in your shoulders.

Roll hips in circles

Place your hands on to your hips, with your feet a shoulder-width apart, roll your hips in one direction and then in the other. As you roll your hips around in a circle, try to make sure the movement is coming from your hips and not from your legs.

Squats

Perform 10–30 squats to feel your whole body loosen up. As you start off with the squats, you can start with half squats and gradually increase into full deep squats.

Calf raises

Perform the calf raises as normal, and really try to stand on your tip-toes to feel your calves.

Step-ups

Perform any type of step-ups until you feel your heart rate increase. This should take no longer than three minutes.

You can now add in stretches if you feel you need to release some muscles, or, if your muscles are ready, you can now start your training session.

When beginning your weight training sessions, do the first exercise with no weight and perform the motion with strict control, normally around 20 reps. Then perform the first set with a light weight. After that, you will be ready to lift heavy weights and get stuck in.

When training with weights, I also try to stretch in between all of my sets. Make sure you're stretching the muscle that you're exercising, as this helps to open up the muscles and to incorporate more of the muscle fibres into the next set. This in turn helps you gain more tone, strength and definition.

COOL-DOWN

The cool-down phase is to make a transition for your muscles, heart and lungs to a resting or near resting state. You should slowly decrease your intensity as you go through your cool-down, which will decrease your heart rate and blood pressure.

CV TRAINING SESSIONS

Once you have finished your training session, slow the pace down gradually until you are either spinning your legs out with no resistance if you are cycling or gradually slow to a walk if you are running. Keep moving at the slower pace until you feel your body relax and your heart rate decrease. Once you feel nice and relaxed and back to some normality you can now perform the stretches.

WEIGHT AND CIRCUIT TRAINING SESSIONS

Complete the cool-down in the same manner as the CV cool-down. Normally when I finish circuit training or weight training, I go for a walk and try to relax my body. I might use some of the warm-up movements to make sure my muscles feel free of lactic acid, such as arm circles.

Once your heart rate has come down, perform the stretches.

WARM-UP AND COOL-DOWN STRETCHES

Try to stretch after the cool-down to make sure you don't ache too much the next day, and to help release the tension from within the muscles.

I used the myo stretch (meaning the muscle stretch) throughout the 12-week programme on a weekly basis to work on specific muscles that felt tight. It is an hour-long stretching routine that encompasses the majority of the muscles within your body.

You can follow this routine (see page XX), or below are a few basic stretches that I would include in my training routine. Do these in between sets and at the end of training sessions.

HOW TO STRETCH

When you stretch, there is no specific time to hold each stretch. Remember one thing though: the smaller the stretch the better, so listen to your body. You need to find a stretch that gives you no burning sensation, shaking within the muscle, or pain, but instead a stretch that is small enough so you can just feel it.

THE STRETCHES

Calf (gastrocnemius) stretch

Place both hands on a wall in front of you. Extend one leg backwards as far as comfortable, keeping it straight and your front leg bent. Make sure your feet are parallel with each other, and push up diagonally into the wall while pressing your heel down into the floor. You should feel a stretch in the back of your lower leg.

 >>

Soleus stretch

Place both hands on a wall in front of you. Extend one leg backwards, and maintain a bend in it. Make sure your feet are parallel with each other, and push up diagonally into the wall while pressing your heel down into the floor. You should feel a stretch deep in the back of your lower leg.

 <<

Hamstring stretch

Stand with one foot on a chair or raised object. Keep your leg slightly bent and your foot flat on the chair. While keeping your back straight, lean forwards from your hip and tilt your bum upwards. You should be able to feel a stretch in the back of your thigh.

>>

Quad stretch

Stand on one leg either balancing or holding on to a wall or object. Keep your whole body straight and your legs in line with each other. Your knees should be together and, holding your foot behind your buttock, tilt your hip forwards. This enhances the stretch on the front of your thigh.

 <<

Adductor stretch

Stand with your feet wide apart. Keep one leg straight with the toes pointing forwards. Bend the other leg and allow your foot to turn outwards to balance you. While in this position, lower your groin towards the ground – to get more of a stretch you can lean your body towards your straight leg. This is not the best adductor stretch, but is good for when you are on the go.

Hip flexor stretch

Extend one leg backwards as far as is comfortable, and keep it bent. Place both feet parallel with each other. Push your pelvis forwards, and lean slightly backwards towards your back leg. If you require, you can support yourself next to a wall or object to balance yourself.

Glute stretch

Lie on your back on the floor face up. Cross one leg over the other leg, and rest your foot on the thigh. Start to bring your foot towards your buttock. Grasp the thigh just under the knee. Pull the leg up and towards your chest.

Abdominal stretch

Lie face down on the floor, keeping your hands in front of you about a shoulder-width apart. Keep your hips, legs and feet flat on the ground. Raise your torso off the ground until your arms are almost straight.

Lower back stretch

Lie on your back, face up. Hold on to the back of your thighs just underneath the knees. Pull your knees towards your chest, allowing your buttocks to rise off the ground.

If you cannot feel the stretch there is an alternative method. Kneel on the ground, with your weight on your heels. Reach forwards with your hands, and let your head relax between your arms.

Lat stretch

Place your feet shoulder-width apart, and extend one arm across your body in front of you. Reach across as far as possible with your hands while leaning slightly forwards. The key is to try and arch the side of your back. You can vary this by holding on to an object or doorway. This will give you a deeper stretch into the lats.

Rhomboid stretch

Place your hands together in front of you at about shoulder height. Reach forwards as far as is comfortable with your hands, trying to round the middle/upper part of your back.

Pectoral stretch

Stand alongside a wall, with your feet shoulder-width apart. Bend your arm to a 90° angle at the elbow, and rest your forearm on to the wall or door frame. At the same time place the same-sided leg forwards. Turn your body and shoulders away from the bent arm until you feel a stretch.

Anterior deltoid stretch

Place your hands into the base of your back. Drop your shoulders forwards and raise your chest up just like you're taking a deep breath. You should feel a stretch at the front of your shoulders.

Deltoid stretch

Place one arm across the front of your body. You can either keep that arm straight or you can bend it to a 90° angle. Pull your arm in and towards the opposite arm until you feel a stretch.

Triceps stretch

Place one hand up and behind your head with your elbow pointing upwards. With your other hand (depending on your flexibility) either pull the elbow down from the top or push the elbow from the front.

Biceps stretch

Hold on to a bench with your hands facing towards your body and your forearms facing away from your body. Keep your arms straight and lean backwards and down until you feel a stretch.

>>

<<

Forearm flexor stretches

With one hand, hold on to the opposite fingers and straighten your arm so your forearm is facing upwards. Then pull your fingers towards your body.

Forearm extensor stretches

With one hand, hold on to the opposite fingers and straighten your arm so your forearm is facing down. Then pull your fingers towards your body.

>>

Trapezius and neck stretch

While looking straight ahead and keeping your head up, allow your head (ear) to drop towards one of your shoulders. Once in this position, pull the opposite shoulder down with your other hand to feel a stretch in your upper trapezius.

<<

NUTRITION PLANS AND TRAINING SESSIONS

06

THE BEGINNING

Front view of me at the beginning of week 1.

Back view of me at the beginning of week 1.

BODYBUILDING POSES

Abdominal pose

Rear double biceps

Front lat spread

Lat spread

HEALTH CHECK AT THE BEGINNING

Throughout the 12 weeks, use the tests and training sessions to monitor your own progress and to help focus on your weaker areas.

MY RESULTS

Statistics	Weight (kg): 87.5
	Height (cm): 175.5
Health tests	BMI: 28.1
	RHR: 79
	BP: 133/92
	Fat (%): 20.9
	Glucose: 5.9
	Cholesterol: 5.9
	Lung function: 600
Measurements (cm)	Neck: 40.64
	Chest: 99.06
	Arms: R: 34.29 L: 34.92
	Navel: 90.17
	Hips: 87.63
	Thighs: R: 60.96 L: 59.69
	Calves: R: 40.64 L: 39.37
Calliper test (mm)	Biceps: 6
	Triceps: 8
	Waist: 15
	Subscapularis: 12
	Total: 41
	Calliper fat (%): 16.6
Fitness tests	Bleep test (level): 10.7
Maximum reps in one minute	Push-ups: 59
	½ sit-ups: 60
	Squats: 52
	Dips: 55
	Max pull-ups: 12
One rep maximum weight training (kg)	Squats: 110
	Bench press: 100
	Military press: 60
	Deadlifts: 120

YOUR RESULTS

Statistics	Weight (kg):
	Height (cm):
Health tests	BMI:
	RHR:
	BP: /
	Fat (%):
	Glucose:
	Cholesterol:
	Lung Function:
Measurements (cm)	Neck:
	Chest:
	Arms: R: L:
	Navel:
	Hips:
	Thighs: R: L:
	Calves: R: L:
Calliper test (mm)	Biceps:
	Triceps:
	Waist:
	Subscapularis:
	Total:
	Calliper fat (%):
Fitness tests	Bleep test (level):
Maximum reps in one minute	Push-ups:
	½ sit-ups:
	Squats:
	Dips:
	Max pull-ups:
One rep maximum weight training (kg)	Squats:
	Bench press:
	Military press:
	Deadlifts:

WEEK ONE NUTRITION PLAN WEEK 1

WEEK 1 OVERVIEW

Day	Breakfast	Lunch	Dinner
1	Muesli with fresh fruit	Smoked salmon pitta	Beef stir fry
2	Fruit porridge	Tuna and olive salad	Chicken with roasted sweet potatoes
3	Fresh fruit and seeds	Tuna salad with sweet potato	Slow roasted orange veal
4	Wheat biscuits or muesli with fruit	Turkey wrap	Jacket potatoes with cheese
5	Fruit salad	Butternut squash and vegetables	Spicy salmon
6	Fruit smoothie 1	Pitta turkey salad	Grilled tandoori chicken
7	Omelette	Butternut squash and coriander soup	Mackerel salad

SHOPPING LIST **WEEK 1**

CARBOHYDRATES
1 bag of brown rice
480g of muesli
1 bag of pine nuts
8 wholemeal/brown pitta breads
240g porridge oats
4 jacket potatoes
1 bag of sunflower seeds
1 bag of pumpkin seeds
9 sweet potatoes
4 organic tortilla wraps
Wheat biscuits

DAIRY AND NON-DAIRY ALTERNATIVES
350g low fat cottage cheese/ soft goat's cheese
8 eggs
40g feta/goat's cheese
1 light soft cheese/soft goat's cheese
680ml skimmed/ soya/rice/ oat milk
2kg soya/plain yoghurt

FISH
8 anchovy fillets
4 mackerel fillets
4 salmon fillets
1 pack of smoked salmon
4 small tuna cans
350g tuna steaks

MEAT
4 200g beef steaks
8 chicken breasts
400g lean ham
8 turkey breasts
1.4kg rack of veal

FRUIT
6 apples
12 bananas
1 punnet of blueberries
2 lemons
2 mangos
1 orange
1 large pineapple
1 punnet of raspberries

VEGETABLES
1 avocado
2 bags of baby spinach
25g black olives
3 butternut squash
5 carrots
2 celery sticks
2 courgettes
1 cucumber
175g French beans
2 leeks
4 lettuces
265g mangetout
150g mushrooms
1 onion
115g plum tomatoes
5 red onions
5 red peppers
20 red tomatoes
100g rocket salad
26 spring onions
1 bag of sweet corn
2 yellow peppers

HERBS
Basil
Black pepper
Chinese five-spice
Coriander
Cumin
Dill
Fresh ginger
1 garlic bulb
Green chilli
Ground coriander
Mint
Nutmeg
Paprika
Turmeric

OTHER
Balsamic vinegar
Beef stock
Corn flour
Chicken stock
Cold-pressed extra virgin olive oil
Ginger wine
Soy sauce
Tandoori paste
Tomato purée

SNACKS
Fruit
Wholegrain crispbread/ crackers/flat breads
Small bowl of muesli
Soya yoghurt
Nuts (cashew, pine or occasionally mixed nuts)
Soya nuts
Seeds (pumpkin or sunflower)

FRUIT DRINKS
1 carton fruit juice drink

RECIPES **WEEK 1** DAY 1

BREAKFAST MUESLI WITH FRESH FRUIT

240g muesli (60g per person)

Serving of milk (soya/rice/oat or skimmed milk)

Fruit of your choice, cut into chunks (1 piece of fruit per person

1 Pour muesli into a bowl, add milk.
2 Serve with fruit.

LUNCH SMOKED SALMON PITTA

4 wholemeal pitta breads (hot or cold)

Smoked salmon

Soft goat's cheese/low fat soft cheese (small serving per person)

2 spring onions, finely sliced

200g baby spinach

4 large tomatoes, sliced into quarters

1 red pepper, finely sliced

1 Cut open the pitta bread and spread the goat's cheese thinly across one side.
2 Add the smoked salmon and sprinkle on the spring onions.
3 Serve with spinach, tomatoes and red pepper.

DINNER BEEF STIR FRY

2 teaspoons corn flour

115ml beef stock

2 tablespoons soy sauce

800g of lean steak

1 tablespoon olive oil

1 garlic clove, finely chopped

2cm piece ginger

150g mushrooms

100g of mangetout

Brown rice

4 spring onions, chopped

1 Blend together the stock, corn flour and soy sauce.
2 Mix the beef, olive oil, garlic and ginger in a large bowl.
3 Heat a large frying pan or wok, and when hot add beef mixture and heat until meat is brown, then set aside.
4 Add the spring onions, mangetout and mushrooms to the hot pan, and fry until slightly crunchy.
5 Add the stock and corn flour mixture to the pan, stir over high heat until sauce has thickened.
6 Add the meat back into the pan, heat and stir well. Serve with brown rice.

RECIPES **WEEK 1** DAY 2

BREAKFAST FRUIT PORRIDGE

240g of porridge oats (60g per person)

2–3 apples, chopped

120ml of water or milk (soya/rice/oat or skimmed milk) – enough to cover the oats and apples

1 Slowly bring the water and/or milk to the boil in a saucepan. Add the oats and chopped apples.

2 Cook for 10 minutes, stirring continuously until thickened. If the mixture becomes too thick, add more water or milk. Serve immediately.

LUNCH TUNA AND OLIVE SALAD

175g French beans, topped and tailed

350g fresh tuna steaks

115g baby plum tomatoes, halved

8 anchovy fillets, drained on kitchen paper

25g stoned black olives in brine, drained

Fresh basil leaves to garnish

For the dressing:

1 tablespoon olive oil

1 garlic clove, crushed

1 tablespoon lemon juice

1 tablespoon basil leaves, shredded

1 Boil the French beans in a small saucepan for 5 minutes, or until slightly tender. Drain and keep warm.

2 Season the tuna steaks with black pepper, and place tuna on grill rack and cook for 4–5 minutes on each side, or until cooked through.

3 Drain the tuna on kitchen paper, and flake the tuna into bite size pieces using a knife and fork.

4 Mix the tuna, French beans, tomatoes, anchovies and olives in a bowl and keep warm.

5 Mix all of the dressing ingredients together and pour over the tuna salad. Garnish with basil and serve.

DINNER CHICKEN WITH ROASTED SWEET POTATOES

3 sweet potatoes, chopped

1 butternut squash, peeled and chopped

1 red onion, peeled and chopped

6 spring onions, finely sliced

40g feta/goat's cheese, cut into small chunks

4 chicken breasts, sliced

2 tablespoons olive oil

1 teaspoon dried basil

1 teaspoon dried basil

1 teaspoon dried basil

3 tomatoes, roughly chopped

Handful of lettuce per person

1 Preheat oven to 190°C (375°F). Place the sweet potatoes and butternut squash into an ovenproof dish and drizzle half of the extra virgin olive oil over the top, mix well. Place into the oven and cook for 35–45 minutes.
2 Meanwhile, heat the rest of the olive oil over a medium heat and cook the chicken breasts for 8–12 minutes, until golden brown and thoroughly cooked.
3 Add the red onion, spring onions, dried basil and tomatoes to the sweet potatoes and butternut squash dish, stir well and cook for a further 5 minutes.
4 Sprinkle the cheese over the top and cook for another 3–4 minutes.
5 Serve the sweet potatoes and butternut squash topped with cheese with the chicken on a bed of lettuce leaves. Decorate with spring onions.

Lunch for tomorrow:
TUNA SALAD WITH SWEET POTATO
Consider preparing extra sweet potatoes in advance for tomorrow's lunch.

RECIPES **WEEK 1** DAY 3

BREAKFAST FRESH FRUIT AND SEEDS

8 tablespoons soya/plain yoghurt

Sprinkle of sunflower or pumpkin seeds

2 pieces of fruit of your choice per person

1 Mix together the soya/plain yoghurt, seeds and fruit.
2 Divide into four portions.

LUNCH TUNA SALAD WITH SWEET POTATO

4 sweet potatoes, cooked (1 per person)

4 small tinned tuna (1 per person)

100g rocket leaves

4 tomatoes, roughly chopped

¼ cucumber, roughly chopped

50g mangetout

1 red pepper, sliced

1 tablespoon balsamic vinegar

1 tablespoon olive oil

1 Preheat oven to 190°C (375°F).
2 Cut the sweet potatoes into small chunks and drizzle with a tablespoon of extra virgin olive oil. Cook in the oven for 30–40 minutes.
3 Place rocket leaves, mangetout, tomatoes, cucumber and red pepper into a salad bowl.
4 Add balsamic vinegar and olive oil and mix well.
5 Serve with tuna, sweet potatoes and salad.

DINNER SLOW ROASTED ORANGE VEAL

1.4kg rack of veal, trim fat

2 carrots, sliced lengthways

2 courgettes, chopped

2 red onions, chopped

2 tablespoons olive oil

4 spring onions, finely chopped

Orange zest, finely grated

60ml of orange juice

For the dressing:

1 butternut squash, peeled and chopped into small pieces

150g low fat natural/soya yoghurt

2 tablespoons fresh mint

½ tablespoon olive oil

2 tablespoons lemon juice

1 Preheat oven to 200°C (400°F). Put butternut squash, carrots, courgettes and onions into a large baking dish. Drizzle over half of the olive oil and mix well.
2 Mix the spring onions, orange zest, orange juice and the rest of the olive oil to make a mixture.
3 Place veal on a wire rack set over vegetables and coat meat with mixture.
4 Roast veal for 40 minutes, or until cooked throughout.
5 Remove meat from oven, cover with foil and rest for 10 minutes.
6 Mix all of the dressing ingredients in a bowl, and serve vegetables and meat with a drizzle of dressing over the top.

Lunch for tomorrow:
TURKEY WRAP
Consider preparing turkey breast in advance for tomorrow's lunch.

RECIPES **WEEK 1** DAY 4

BREAKFAST WHEAT BISCUITS OR MUESLI WITH FRUIT

560ml milk (soya/rice/oat or skimmed milk)

2–3 wheat biscuits or 240g of muesli (60g per person)

1 piece of fruit of your choice

1 Place your choice of cereal in a bowl and add milk.
2 Serve with fruit.

LUNCH TURKEY WRAP

4 turkey breasts, cooked and sliced

4 organic wholewheat wraps, serve hot or cold

200g mixed salad

4–5 tomatoes, sliced

1 red onion, finely chopped

1 yellow pepper, sliced

4 tablespoons of soya/plain yoghurt

1 Heat some extra virgin olive oil (½ tablespoon) in a frying pan over a medium heat.
2 Slice and cook 4 turkey breasts (1 per person) until golden.
3 Place the salad, red onion, tomatoes, yellow pepper and cooked turkey breasts into a salad bowl and mix well.
4 Drizzle over the yoghurt and add the salad to the wrap and roll up.

DINNER JACKET POTATOES WITH COTTAGE OR GOAT'S CHEESE

4 large baking potatoes (cut a cross in the centre of each potato and prick the skins with a fork)

3 teaspoons sun-dried tomato purée

½ teaspoon ground coriander

1 tablespoon olive oil

4 spring onions, finely chopped

1 fresh green chilli, deseeded and finely chopped

1 tablespoon fresh coriander

350g low fat cottage cheese/ soft goat's cheese

Handful of pine nuts

Side salad:

Generous amounts of mixed salad leaves

4 large tomatoes, chopped

1 red pepper, chopped

¼ cucumber, chopped

1 Preheat oven to 200°C (400°F). Bake the potatoes for one hour, or until soft and cooked. Meanwhile prepare the salad.
2 Mix the sun-dried tomato purée and ground coriander together in a bowl.
3 Just before the potatoes are ready, heat the olive oil in a small saucepan and add the spring onions and chopped chillies and cook for 2–3 minutes, stirring occasionally until soft.
4 Stir in the sun-dried tomato paste and cook for a further 1 minute. Remove from heat and stir in the chopped coriander.
5 Place the cheese in a bowl and stir in the tomato mixture.
6 Divide the cheese mixture equally among the potatoes.
7 Serve with salad and add a sprinkle of pine nuts over the top.

**Lunch for tomorrow:
BUTTERNUT SQUASH AND VEGETABLES**
See the following page and consider preparing your lunch in advance.

RECIPES **WEEK 1** DAY 5

BREAKFAST FRUIT SALAD

8 tablespoons soya/plain yoghurt (2 tablespoons per person)

80g oats

60g sunflower seeds or pumpkin seeds

4–5 pieces of fruit (preferably ones in season)

1 Dice fruit into chunks and divide into four portions.
2 Add 2 tablespoons of soya/plain yoghurt to each portion and sprinkle with oats and seeds.

LUNCH BUTTERNUT SQUASH AND VEGETABLES

1 butternut squash, peeled and chopped

2 sweet potatoes, peeled, and diced into cubes

1 leek, chopped

1 red onion, quartered

1 tablespoon, olive oil

Handful of coriander, chopped

Handful of rocket leaves per person

For the dressing:

¼ grated cucumber

4 tablespoons soya/plain yoghurt

1 tablespoon olive oil

1 teaspoon balsamic vinegar

2 teaspoons black pepper

2 teaspoons dried dill

1 Preheat the oven to 190°C (375°F). Place the butternut squash, sweet potatoes, onion and leek into a large baking dish. Drizzle with olive oil and season with black pepper and coriander.

2 Cook for 30–40 minutes, or until vegetables are cooked. Stir if necessary.

3 Meanwhile, place all dressing ingredients into a small bowl and mix well.

4 Remove from the oven and serve with rocket leaves, and drizzle the dressing over the top.

DINNER SPICY SALMON

4 Salmon fillets

2 teaspoons Chinese five-spice powder

2.5cm ginger, cut into thin strips

2 tablespoons ginger wine

2 tablespoons soy sauce

1 tablespoon olive oil

Brown rice

Side vegetables:

1 leek, finely shredded

1 carrot, sliced lengthways

115g mangetout, cut into thin strips

1 Rub Chinese five-spice powder into both sides of the salmon fillets.

2 Place vegetables into a bowl, and add ginger wine and soy sauce.

3 Preheat the grill to a medium heat. Boil water and add the rice.

4 Place the salmon fillets on the grill and brush with some soy sauce. Cook for a few minutes on each side.

5 Meanwhile, heat the olive oil in wok or frying pan and stir fry vegetables for 3–5 minutes.

6 When the vegetables and salmon are cooked, transfer to plates and serve with brown rice.

**Marinade for tomorrow's dinner:
GRILLED TANDOORI CHICKEN**
Consider preparing marinade for tomorrow's dinner in advance (leave in fridge overnight).

RECIPES **WEEK 1** DAY 6

BREAKFAST FRUIT SMOOTHIE 1

2 large mangos, peeled and chopped
4 bananas, chopped
2 handfuls of raspberries

1 Blend mangos, bananas and raspberries, and serve.

LUNCH PITTA TURKEY SALAD

4 wholemeal pitta breads
4 turkey breasts, cooked and sliced
Generous amount of salad leaves
1 avocado, sliced
1 red pepper, sliced
1 yellow pepper, sliced
2 spring onions, finely chopped
½ tablespoon olive oil
4 tablespoons of soya/plain yoghurt

1 Place the salad leaves, avocado, peppers and chopped spring onions in a salad bowl and mix.
2 Slice open the pitta bread and fill with turkey, salad and a dollop of soya/plain yoghurt.
3 Serve immediately.

DINNER GRILLED TANDOORI CHICKEN

100g natural soya/plain yoghurt
4 chicken breasts, diced
300g spinach
1 handful of coriander, chopped
8–10 tablespoons of sweetcorn
Brown rice
For the marinade:
1 tablespoon tandoori paste
1 teaspoon cumin
300g natural soya/plain yoghurt
1 tablespoon lemon juice
1 garlic glove, crushed

1 In a bowl, add the marinade ingredients together and mix well.
2 Add the diced chicken and coat with marinade. Leave in the fridge for at least 2–3 hours.
3 Preheat grill to a medium heat and cover a baking tray with baking paper.
4 Skewer the chicken and place on to a baking tray. Grill for 8–12 minutes, or until chicken is cooked (keep turning).
5 Boil the rice and add the sweetcorn for the last 2 minutes.
6 Serve the chicken, spinach, sweetcorn and rice. Pour the remaining yoghurt over the top and garnish with coriander.

RECIPES **WEEK 1** DAY 7

BREAKFAST OMELETTE

8 eggs (2 eggs per person)
4 tablespoons of cold water
8 teaspoons of extra virgin olive oil
400g lean ham
1 courgette, finely sliced
4 spring onions, finely chopped

1 Cook one omelette at a time, beat the eggs with some water in a bowl.
2 Heat the extra virgin olive oil in a non-stick pan over a high heat and pour in the eggs. Cook for 2 minutes, or until the mixture just begins to set.
3 Place ham and courgette on top of the egg mixture and cook until the omelette has set.
4 Sprinkle on the spring onions, fold omelette in half, and serve.

LUNCH BUTTERNUT SQUASH AND CORIANDER SOUP

900ml of chicken stock
1kg butternut squash, peeled and chopped
1 onion, roughly chopped
2 carrots, roughly chopped
2 celery sticks, roughly chopped
1 garlic clove, crushed
1 teaspoon paprika
½ teaspoon turmeric
½ teaspoon ground coriander
½ teaspoon ground nutmeg

1 In a large saucepan bring chicken stock to the boil. Add the vegetables and spices and bring back to the boil.
2 Reduce heat and simmer for 20 minutes, or until vegetables are soft.
3 Allow to cool and serve.

DINNER MACKEREL SALAD

4 cooked mackerel, skin removed
Generous amount of mixed salad leaves
1 red pepper, sliced and deseeded
4–5 tomatoes, sliced
¼ cucumber, sliced
For the dressing:
3 tablespoons of soya/plain yoghurt
Pine nuts, small sprinkle
½ tablespoon balsamic vinegar
Black pepper

1 Place mixed salad leaves, peppers, tomatoes and cucumber on a plate.
2 Cut the mackerel into pieces and place on top of salad.
3 To make the dressing, mix the yoghurt, pine nuts and balsamic vinegar in a small bowl and add black pepper to taste. Add dressing to salad.

Lunch for tomorrow:
BEETROOT SALAD
Consider preparing rice and shallots in advance for tomorrow's lunch (see page 97).

TRAINING DIARY **WEEK 1**

WEEK 1 OVERVIEW
Day 1: Weights – Upper body
Day 2: Rest
Day 3: CV – Run; PT – Upper body
Day 4: Rest
Day 5: Rest
Day 6: Rest
Day 7: Circuits; Myo Stretch

MY DIARY

Day 1 (Monday)
I tried to shave last night with an epilator but I only did one strip on my lower leg, it was so painful I had to give up. Never again. First day in and enjoyed my training but had a shaving rash on my legs.
Tiredness 7
Stress 7
Sleep 8 hours

Day 2 (Tuesday)
Aching over my upper body, which is called DOMS (delayed onset muscle soreness), but it is a good ache that tells me that I have been working hard.
Tiredness 6
Stress 6
Sleep 7 hours 30 minutes

Day 3 (Wednesday)
No aches or pains today, but when I got back from my first run I ended up getting blisters and sore feet.
Tiredness 4
Stress 9
Sleep 3 hours 45 minutes

Day 4 (Thursday)
It actually feels like I have lost weight, but I'm not going to weigh myself until Sunday as I don't want to be disappointed. I managed to have a myo massage today to get into my muscles and release any dysfunctions I have in them. I was also using this massage to counteract my postural concerns.
Tiredness 8
Stress 7
Sleep 8 hours

Day 5 (Friday)
Going to London today for work, so I will have to train either in my room or outside. I am now really looking forwards to training all the time.
Tiredness 7
Stress 6
Sleep 7 hours 30 minutes

Day 6 (Saturday)
For some reason I was very hungry today, and so I drank a little more water to suppress the hunger until dinner. Came back from London for my photos and results tomorrow.
Tiredness 5
Stress 4
Sleep 5 hours 30 minutes

Day 7 (Sunday)
It was good to do my tests today to compare my results from when I started. Not only were my results looking good, but my stomach wasn't so bloated, my athletes foot wasn't itchy anymore, and my spots started to dry up and disappear. I did the 1-hour myo stretch today and I will be doing it every Sunday from now on, as I felt so good afterwards.
Tiredness 6
Stress 5
Sleep 4 hours 30 minutes

TRAINING SESSION **WEEK 1** DAY 1

MY TRAINING SESSION

AM Rest

PM Training session Weights – Upper body

Time trained 7.00–8.20 p.m.

Session time 1 hour 20 minutes

RPE 3/10

WORKOUT
Incline bench press
1 × 20 warm-up – with just Olympic bar
Set and Rep: 1. 20   2. 10   3. 10   4. 10   5. 10
Weight (kg): N/A   40   50   60   60

Military press
Set and Rep: 1. 10   2. 10   3. 7   4. 8
Weight (kg): 25   30   40   35

Deadlifts
Set and Rep: 1. 10   2. 10   3. 10   4. 10
Weight (kg): 60   80   80   90

Arm curl (Olympic bar)
Set and Rep: 1. 10   2. 10
Weight (kg): 30   30

My notes: I was feeling sore from yesterday's test day. My chest, quads, adductors, hamstrings and triceps were the main muscles that were sore. So I took this session easy today, to re-teach my muscles and also to see what I could lift comfortably with good technique.

I didn't do any triceps exercises due to them already feeling fairly pumped after the two compound exercises.

YOUR TRAINING SESSION

AM

PM Training session Weights – Upper body

Time trained

Session time

RPE   /10

WORKOUT
Incline bench press
1 × 20 warm-up – with just Olympic bar
Set and Rep: 1.   2.   3.   4.   5.
Weight (kg): N/A

Military press
Set and Rep: 1.   2.   3.   4.
Weight (kg):

Deadlifts
Set and Rep: 1.   2.   3.   4.
Weight (kg):

Arm curl (Olympic bar)
Set and Rep: 1.   2.
Weight (kg):

Your notes:

TRAINING SESSION **WEEK 1** DAY 3

MY TRAINING SESSION

AM Rest

PM Training session CV – Run

Time trained 6.45–7.15 p.m.

Session time 30 minutes

RPE 5/10

PM Training session PT – Upper body

Time trained 7.15–7.45 p.m.

Session time 30 minutes

RPE 4/10

WORKOUT
Once you have finished the 3-mile run try to go straight into the PT.

Run
Actual distance: 3.1 miles
Run time: 30 minutes
Average pace: 10 m/m

PT – Upper body
No rest in between sets and reps.
Regular pull-ups: 1–6 and 6–1
Total: 42

YOUR TRAINING SESSION

AM

PM Training session CV – Run

Time trained

Session time

RPE /10

PM Training session PT – Upper body

Time trained

Session time

RPE /10

WORKOUT

Run
Actual distance: miles
Run time: minutes
Average pace: m/m

PT – Upper body
No rest in between sets and reps.
Regular pull-ups:
Total:

Regular press-ups: 1–10 and 10 –1
Total: 110

Crunches: 3 × 30
Leg levers: 3 × 15

My notes: I choose to do a really slow and easy run due to not having run or trained for over 4 months. I also ache slightly on my chest today, which is the DOMS.

Regular press-ups:
Total:

Crunches: 3 ×
Leg levers: 3 ×

Your notes:

TRAINING SESSION **WEEK 1** DAY 7

MY TRAINING SESSION

AM Rest

PM **Training session** Circuits

Time trained 7.00–8.20 p.m.

Session time 1 hour 20 minutes

RPE 7/10

WORKOUT
Complete the first set in each exercise for cycle 1 and cycle 2, and then move on to the next set for cycle 1 and 2. Repeat until you have completed all six sets in the first and second cycles.

YOUR TRAINING SESSION

AM

PM **Training session** Circuits

Time trained

Session time

RPE   /10

WORKOUT

CYCLE 1
Pull-ups
Set and Rep: 1. 15   2. 13   3. 11   4. 9   5. 7   6. 4
Incline press
Set and Rep: 1. 30   2. 28   3. 26   4. 24   5. 22   6. 20
Weight (kg):   30   30   30   30   30   30

CYCLE 2
Burpees
Set and Rep: 1. 15   2. 13   3. 11   4. 9   5. 7   6. 4
Squat thrusts
Set and Rep: 1. 15   2. 13   3. 11   4. 9   5. 7   6. 4
Alternate squat thrusts
Set and Rep: 1. 15   2. 13   3. 11   4. 9   5. 7   6. 4

Complete all three sets in a row for the first exercise for each exercise. No rest between sets and exercises.

CYCLE 3
Lat raise, weight 17.5lb: 3×15
Jump over (hands on floor): 3×15
Lat pull-downs (close grip), weight 30kg: 3×15
Wide squat thrusts: 3×15
Bench press, weight 35kg: 3×15
Squat jumps: 3×15

Superset

	Upright row			Dumbbell press		
Sets and Rep	1. 10	2. 10	3. 10	1. 10	2. 10	3. 10
Weight (kg)	30	30	30	35	35	35

Superset

	Arm curl (Olympic bar)			Triceps press-down (cable)		
Sets and Reps	1. 10	2. 10	3. 10	1. 15	2. 12	3. 12
Weight (kg)	30	30	30	30	30	30

CYCLE 1
Pull-ups
Set and Rep: 1.   2.   3.   4.   5.   6.
Incline press
Set and Rep: 1.   2.   3.   4.   5.   6.
Weight (kg):

CYCLE 2
Burpees
Set and Rep: 1.   2.   3.   4.   5.   6.
Squat thrusts
Set and Rep: 1.   2.   3.   4.   5.   6.
Alternate squat thrusts
Set and Rep: 1.   2.   3.   4.   5.   6.

CYCLE 3
Lat raise, weight   kg: $3 \times$
Jump over (hands on floor): $3 \times$
Lat pull-downs (close grip), weight   kg: $3 \times$
Wide squat thrusts: $3 \times$
Bench press, weight   kg: $3 \times$
Squat jumps: $3 \times$

Superset

	Upright row			Dumbbell press		
Set and Rep:	1.	2.	3.	1.	2.	3.
Weight (kg):						

Superset

	Arm curl (Olympic bar)			Triceps press-down (cable)		
Set and Rep:	1.	2.	3.	1.	2.	3.
Weight (kg):						

Your notes:

WEEK 1 TESTS

Take a photo of yourself from front and back to help gauge your progress.

Front view of me at the end of week 1.

Back view of me at the end of week 1.

MY WEEKLY TESTS

Weight (kg): 85.5
Height (cm): 175.5
BMI: 27.8
RHR: 74
BP: 137/89
Fat %: 18.7

Measurements (cm)
Neck: 40
Chest: 100.96
Arm: R 34.29   L 34.29
Navel: 87.63
Hips: 88.90
Thighs: R 60.96   L 59.69
Calves: R 40.64   L 39.37

YOUR WEEKLY TESTS

Weight (kg):
Height (cm):
BMI:
RHR:
BP:
Fat %:

Measurements (cm)
Neck:
Chest:
Arm: R   L
Navel:
Hips:
Thighs: R   L
Calves: R   L

WEEK **TWO** NUTRITION PLAN **WEEK 2**

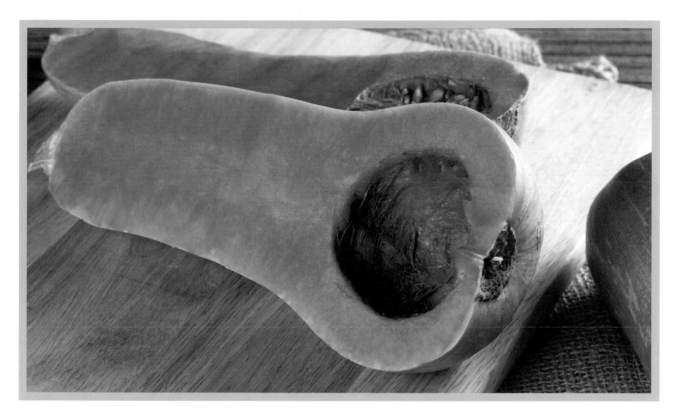

WEEK 2 OVERVIEW

Day	Breakfast	Lunch	Dinner
1	Fruit salad	Beetroot salad	Lamb ratatouille
2	Muesli with fresh fruit	Lamb with feta/goat's cheese	Chilli fish
3	Scrambled eggs with wild mushrooms	Tuna salad with sweet potato	Turkey stir fry with orange
4	Fruit porridge	Vegetable soup	Tuna steak and cannellini bean salad
5	Fresh fruit and seeds	Beef salad pitta	Tandoori turkey salad
6	Fruit smoothie 1	Bean salad	Swordfish with Mediterranean vegetables
7	Omelette	Tuna and olive salad	Hot bean soup with butternut squash

SHOPPING LIST WEEK 2

CARBOHYDRATES
1 bag of brown rice
400g cannellini beans
50g tinned chickpeas
250g couscous
475g kidney beans
490g muesli
10 new potatoes
1 bag of pine nuts
400g pinto beans
8 wholemeal or brown
Pitta breads
320g porridge oats
1 bag of sunflower seeds
1 bag of pumpkin seeds
8 sweet potatoes
4 bags of wild rice

DAIRY AND NON-DAIRY ALTERNATIVES
20 eggs
40g feta/goat's cheese
1520ml skimmed/soya/rice/ oat milk
2kg soya yoghurt

FISH
8 anchovy fillets
4 plaice fillets
200g (× 4) swordfish
4 small tuna cans
750g tuna steaks

MEAT
400g cooked roast beef
6 lamb chops
400g lean ham
8 turkey breasts

FRUIT
7 apples
2 apricots
6 bananas
1 punnet of blueberries
2 lemons
1 lime
2 mangoes
1 orange
2 peaches
1 large pineapple
1 punnet of raspberries

VEGETABLES
2 avocados
4 baby aubergines
2 bags of baby spinach
4 cooked beetroots
25g black olives
175g broccoli
250g cherry tomatoes
1 butternut squash
6 carrots
4 celery sticks
5 courgettes
1 cucumber
175g French beans
2 leeks
3 lettuces
50g mangetout
8 mushrooms
3 onions
135g plum tomatoes
2 red onions
8 red peppers
10 red tomatoes
100g rocket salad
10 spring onions
4 shallots
1 bag of sweet corn
1 yellow pepper

HERBS
Basil
Black pepper
Cayenne pepper
Chilli powder
Chinese five-spice
Chives
Coriander
Coriander seeds
Cumin
Fresh ginger
Garam masala
1 garlic bulb
Ground coriander
Ground pepper
Mint
Parsley
1 red chilli
Rosemary
Turmeric

OTHER
Balsamic vinegar
Chicken stock
Chilli sauce
Cold-pressed extra virgin olive oil
Corn flour
Dijon mustard
Ginger wine
Muscovado sugar
Soy sauce
Sesame oil
Tandoori paste
Tomato purée
Vegetable stock
White wine vinegar
Wholegrain mustard

SNACKS
Fruit
Wholegrain crispbread/ crackers
Flat breads
Small bowl of muesli
Yoghurt/soya yoghurt
Nuts (cashew, pine or occasionally mixed nuts)
Soya nuts
Seeds (pumpkin or sunflower)

FRUIT DRINKS
1 carton fruit juice

RECIPES **WEEK 2** DAY 1

BREAKFAST FRUIT SALAD

See page 85

LUNCH BEETROOT SALAD

100g brown rice

100g wild rice

4 shallots, peeled and halved

2 teaspoons olive oil

4 beetroot, finely diced cooked

Juice of 1 lemon

2 tablespoons fresh mint, chopped

2 tablespoons fresh chives, chopped

1 Preheat oven to 200°C (400°F). Place brown/ wild rice in medium saucepan of water, bring to boil and simmer for 20–30 minutes.
2 Put the shallots on a baking tray, drizzle with olive oil and roast for 8–10 minutes.
3 Drain the rice and allow to cool. Gently mix together the beetroot, lemon juice and mint.
4 Stir in shallots and chives and serve.

DINNER LAMB RATATOUILLE

8 lamb steaks, lean diced

1 tablespoon olive oil

250g couscous

Spices:

1 tablespoon pepper, freshly ground

2 teaspoons coriander seeds, whole

1 teaspoon garam masala

1 teaspoon chilli powder

For the ratatouille:

2 teaspoons olive oil

4 baby aubergines

1 onion, finely chopped

1 clove garlic, chopped

1 red pepper, deseeded and sliced

1 courgette, sliced

115ml chicken stock

2 tomatoes

1 tablespoon parsley, chopped

1 Mix all the spices in a bowl and brush the steaks with a little olive oil and coat with spice mixture, cover with cling film and refrigerate for 1 hour.
2 To make ratatouille, heat the olive oil in a large frying pan over medium heat.
3 Add aubergines and cook for 4 minutes or until golden. Then add the onion and garlic and cook until lightly coloured.
4 Next add the red pepper and courgette and cook for a further minute. Then pour on the chicken stock and add the tomatoes and bring to boil. Cook for a further 5 minutes, add parsley and season to taste.
5 Bring water to the boil and add the couscous, cover with a lid and allow to settle.
6 Heat oil in a frying pan over high heat and cook lamb for 3 minutes on each side.
7 Serve the lamb with ratatouille and couscous.

Lunch for tomorrow:
LAMB RATATOUILLE
Save some lamb ratatouille for tomorrow's lunch.

RECIPES **WEEK 2** DAY 2

BREAKFAST MUESLI WITH FRESH FRUIT

See page 80

LUNCH LAMB WITH FETA/ GOAT'S CHEESE

4 pitta breads, 1 per person (serve hot or cold)

Ratatouille and sauce from last night's dinner

Lettuce

Feta/goat's cheese, small amount

Soya/plain yoghurt

1 Slice open pitta bread and fill with lamb, ratatouille, lettuce and sprinkle with feta/goat's cheese.
2 Drizzle the soya/plain yoghurt over the top.

DINNER CHILLI FISH

4 plaice fillets

1 tablespoon olive oil

1 tablespoon fresh coriander

2 tablespoons lime juice

300ml water

1 tablespoon chilli sauce

2 tablespoons tomato purée

1cm ginger, grated

1 teaspoon muscovado sugar

Lemon wedges, to serve

1 tablespoon white wine vinegar

Brown rice

1 Place fish in a dish, add olive oil, coriander and lime juice and coat well. Cover in cling film and place in the fridge to marinate.
2 Preheat the grill to medium heat. Place water, tomato purée, chilli sauce, white wine vinegar, ginger and sugar in small saucepan. Stir and simmer for 5–8 minutes or until thick.
3 Meanwhile, remove the fish from the marinade and cook under the grill for 5–8 minutes or until the flesh flakes easily.
4 Transfer fish to plates and spoon over the sauce.
5 Serve with brown rice and garnish with lemon wedges.

Lunch for tomorrow:
TUNA SALAD WITH SWEET POTATO
Consider preparing sweet potatoes in advance for tomorrow's lunch.

RECIPES **WEEK 2** DAY 3

BREAKFAST SCRAMBLED EGGS WITH WILD MUSHROOMS

8 wild mushrooms, large

8 eggs

200ml serving of milk
(soya/rice/oat or skimmed milk)

1 tablespoon chives, chopped

2 teaspoons olive oil

Ground black pepper

1 Preheat the grill to high heat. Brush mushrooms with olive oil and season with pepper. Grill for about 10 minutes or until tender.
2 Meanwhile, in a bowl lightly whisk eggs and milk together and lightly season with black pepper.
3 Heat a non-stick frying pan over medium heat and pour in the egg mixture and cook. Keep stirring until the egg is cooked, then stir in chives. Place eggs on the mushrooms and serve.

LUNCH TUNA SALAD WITH SWEET POTATO

See page 83

DINNER TURKEY STIR FRY WITH ORANGE

4 turkey breasts, sliced

1 tablespoon of sesame oil

1 tablespoon olive oil

2 large carrots, thinly sliced

175g small florets of broccoli

2 teaspoons ginger, crushed

2 teaspoons garlic, crushed

4 spring onions, finely sliced

1 tablespoon corn flour

For the marinade:

1 tablespoon wholegrain mustard

2 red peppers, sliced

2 tablespoons soy sauce

1 large orange, finely grated and juiced

Brown rice

1 Marinade: mix together the soy sauce, mustard, orange rind and juice into a small bowl. Stir in the turkey and set aside to marinade. Boil the rice.
2 Heat the olive and sesame oil in a wok or large frying pan over a high heat. Add the carrots and broccoli and cook for 3 minutes.
3 Remove the turkey from mix and add to the wok. Add the garlic, ginger, spring onions and red pepper and stir fry for another 4 minutes.
4 Mix the corn flour and the reserve of the marinade to make a smooth sauce and pour over the turkey.
5 Stir fry for a further 1–2 minutes until the broccoli is tender, serve immediately with brown rice.

Lunch for tomorrow:
VEGRTABLE SOUP
Consider preparing your lunch in advance.

RECIPES **WEEK 2** DAY 4

BREAKFAST FRUIT PORRIDGE

See page 81

LUNCH VEGETABLE SOUP

1 litre vegetable stock

2 carrots, sliced

2 celery sticks, chopped

1 onion, chopped

1 tablespoon fresh parsley, chopped

400g tinned tomatoes

1 tablespoon basil, chopped

1 tablespoon rosemary, finely chopped

1 Bring stock to boil in a large saucepan.
2 Add the carrots, celery, onion, parsley and tomatoes and simmer gently for 30 minutes.
3 Stir through basil and rosemary, and season with black pepper.

DINNER TUNA STEAK AND CANNELLINI BEAN SALAD

1 tablespoon pine nuts

4 × 100g tuna steaks

½ tablespoon olive oil

1 garlic clove, crushed

400g white cannellini beans, drained and rinsed

1 tablespoon basil, finely sliced

½ tablespoon parsley

2 spring onions, finely sliced

Generous amount of mixed salad leaves

1 Heat a small non-stick frying pan over medium heat, add the pine nuts and stir until toasted and golden, then set aside.
2 Heat a large non-stick frying pan over high heat and add the olive oil.
3 Place tuna steaks in frying pan and cook for 2–3 minutes each side. The tuna should still be a little pink in middle. Allow to cool slightly.
4 Place the remaining ingredients and pine nuts in bowl and mix.
5 Serve the tuna with bean salad on the side.

Dinner for tomorrow:
TANDOORI TURKEY SALAD
Consider marinating the turkey overnight for tomorrow's dinner.

RECIPES **WEEK 2** DAY 5

BREAKFAST FRESH FRUIT AND SEEDS

See page 82

LUNCH BEEF SALAD PITTA

4 wholemeal pitta breads (serve hot or cold)

400g cold roast beef, finely sliced

Green salad, generous amounts of

4 large tomatoes, sliced

1 red pepper, sliced

½ red onion, finely sliced

2 tablespoons chopped basil

For the dressing:

2 tablespoons olive oil

1 tablespoon balsamic vinegar

1 teaspoon Dijon mustard

Season with black pepper

1 In a small bowl mix together all the dressing ingredients.
2 Put the remaining ingredients in a large salad bowl and mix well.
3 Slice open the pitta bread and fill with beef and salad.
4 Pour the dressing over the top.

DINNER TANDOORI TURKEY SALAD

4 sweet potatoes, peeled and chopped

½ tablespoon olive oil

400g turkey breasts

100g baby spinach

4 plum tomatoes, thinly sliced

½ cucumber

Coriander, small handful

Lemon wedges

For the marinade:

1 tablespoon tandoori paste

50g of soya/plain yoghurt

For the dressing:

150g of soya/plain yoghurt

2 tablespoons fresh mint

½ tablespoon olive oil

2 tablespoons lemon juice

1 Mix the tandoori paste and yoghurt in a bowl.
2 Add the turkey and coat thoroughly. Cover and chill for 30 minutes – leave overnight if you have time.
3 Meanwhile, preheat the oven to 190°C (375°F).
4 Place sweet potatoes in an ovenproof dish and drizzle with olive oil. Cook for 20–30 minutes or until soft.
5 Preheat grill and cook turkey over a medium heat for 6 minutes each side or until cooked. Remove from the heat and let turkey rest for 5 minutes then slice the turkey into strips.
6 Place the spinach, tomatoes and cucumber in large salad bowl and put turkey strips over the top.
7 Mix the dressing ingredients together in a small bowl and drizzle the dressing over salad.
8 Garnish with coriander and lemon wedges and serve.

Lunch for tomorrow:
BEAN SALAD
Consider preparing eggs in advance (refrigerate overnight).

RECIPES **WEEK 2** DAY 6

BREAKFAST FRUIT SMOOTHIE 1   *See page 87*

LUNCH BEAN SALAD

4 eggs

2 avocados, stoned and peeled

400g tinned kidney beans

400g tinned pinto beans

1 red onion, finely sliced

Coriander, large handful chopped

250g cherry tomatoes, halved

For the dressing:

1 red chilli, finely sliced

½ teaspoon ground cumin

1 tablespoon of lime juice

3 tablespoons olive oil

1 Boil eggs for 6½ minutes, then place in cold water to cool.
2 Slice avocados and place in bowl with the beans, onions, coriander and tomatoes.
3 Mix the dressing ingredients in a small bowl.
4 Once eggs have cooled but are still warm, peel off shells and cut into quarters.
5 Mix the salad with the dressing and place the eggs on top and serve.

DINNER SWORDFISH WITH MEDITERRANEAN VEGETABLES

2 tablespoons olive oil

1 clove of garlic, chopped

2 teaspoons balsamic vinegar

1 tablespoon parsley, chopped

1 tablespoon basil

Juice of ½ lemon

4 x 200g swordfish steaks

1 red pepper, sliced and deseeded

1 yellow pepper, sliced and deseeded

2 courgettes, sliced

1 red onion, sliced

10 new potatoes, thinly sliced

Lemon wedges

1 Preheat the grill to high.
2 Add new potatoes in a baking tray and drizzle with olive oil. Place under the grill for 10–15 minutes.
3 Add the peppers, courgettes and onion into a bowl with half the olive oil and mix.
4 Transfer vegetables to the grill with the new potatoes and cook for 3–5 minutes, turning occasionally until slightly charred.
5 Place cooked vegetables and potatoes into a bowl.
6 To make the mixture for the fish, add garlic, balsamic vinegar, parsley, basil, lemon juice and rest of olive oil and mix together in another bowl.
7 Place fish in foil, add the mixture and wrap.
8 Grill the fish for 2–3 minutes each side or until cooked.
9 Divide vegetables and new potatoes between four plates and place fish on top.
10 Garnish with lemon wedges and serve immediately.

RECIPES **WEEK 2** DAY 7

BREAKFAST OMELETTE   *See page 88*

LUNCH TUNA AND OLIVE SALAD   *See page 81*

DINNER HOT BEAN SOUP WITH
BUTTERNUT SQUASH

1–2 tablespoons olive oil

1 medium onion, chopped and peeled

2 cloves of garlic, peeled and finely chopped

1 butternut squash, peeled and
chopped small

2 large carrots, peeled and chopped

2 celery sticks, trimmed and chopped

1 large courgette, sliced

2 red peppers, deseeded and chopped

1.5 litres (2.5 pints) vegetable stock

50g tinned chickpeas

75g red tinned kidney beans

1 teaspoon cayenne pepper

1 teaspoon turmeric powder

1 Heat the olive oil in large pan over medium heat, add onion and garlic and cook for 2–3 minutes.
2 Add cayenne pepper and turmeric and stir for 2 minutes.
3 Add butternut squash, carrots and celery and cook for a further 4–5 minutes.
4 Next add the courgette and peppers and cook for 2 minutes.
5 Add in the chickpeas, kidney beans, butternut squash and vegetable stock.
6 Cover the pan with lid and simmer gently for 40 minutes to 1 hour.

Lunch for tomorrow:
CHICKEN WRAP
Consider preparing chicken in advance (refrigerate overnight).

TRAINING DIARY **WEEK 2**

WEEK 2 OVERVIEW
Day 1: CV – Row/Cycle
Day 2: Rest
Day 3: Rest
Day 4: PT – Upper body
Day 5: Rest
Day 6: Weights – Upper body
Day 7: CV – Run; Myo stretch

MY DIARY
Day 1 (Monday)
Very busy day today, finished late so ended up eating out at 9.00 p.m., but I did manage to fit in a training session at a local gym which I got for free. I have noticed that my athletes' foot has really started to clear up.
Tiredness 6
Stress 5
Sleep 6 hours 45 minutes

Day 2 (Tuesday)
Finished late again at work and ate out again at 8.00 p.m., all I did was choose the same meal that I would have had if I was making my own meal following the nutrition plan. Shaving rash has stopped hurting and being itchy but it is still there.
Tiredness 6
Stress 5
Sleep 6 hours 45 minutes

Day 3 (Wednesday)
Finished late again, but I met up with my two brothers in central London and had a few drinks (two pints of Guinness and two vodka and diet mixers) with them, then eventually had some food at 9.00 p.m. Stayed out late until 3.30 a.m.
Tiredness 8
Stress 5
Sleep 6 hours

Day 4 (Thursday)
It was hard getting up this morning and even harder to motivate myself to train, but I did and when I finished it was worth it.
Tiredness 9
Stress 6
Sleep 3 hours 30 minutes

Day 5 (Friday)
I was so busy that I found it hard to stop and have lunch so I had it on the move.
Tiredness 7
Stress 7
Sleep 7 hours 15 minutes

Day 6 (Saturday)
I worked until 4.30 p.m. today, but when I finished I managed to fit in a weights session as well as see Alison. I feel as though my chest is getting bigger and stronger.
Tiredness 6
Stress 5
Sleep 4 hours 45 minutes

Day 7 (Sunday)
Finished my tests and photos and had enough time to fit in a three-mile run before going back to London for work. I did, however, go out for a staff party when I was back in London and got back at 1.00 a.m.
Tiredness 6
Stress 6
Sleep 4 hours

TRAINING SESSION **WEEK 2** DAY 1

MY TRAINING SESSION

AM Rest

PM Training session CV– Row/Cycle

Time trained 7.40–8.10 p.m.

Session time 30 minutes

RPE 7/10

WORKOUT
Row – 7500m
Distance: 2500m
Level: 7
Time: 10.04
Stretch and hydrate for five minutes, then straight back into rowing.
Distance: 5000m
Level: 10
Time: 29.56

My notes: I was working away in London so I couldn't get on my bike, which I had planned to do. Instead I managed to get into a gym for free, and use a concept II rowing machine.

At the end of this session I stretched for about 20 minutes because of yesterday's stretching class as I didn't want to lose the effects.

YOUR TRAINING SESSION

AM

PM Training session Row/Cycle

Time trained

Session time

RPE   /10

WORKOUT
Row
Distance: m
Level:
Time:

Distance: m
Level (rowing):
Time:

Or cycle
Distance: miles
Average speed:
Time:

Your notes:

TRAINING SESSION **WEEK 2** DAY 4

MY TRAINING SESSION

AM Rest

PM **Training session** PT – Upper body

Time trained 8.00–8.40 p.m.

Session time 40 minutes

RPE 6/10

WORKOUT

These two cycles work your chest, abs, arms and legs. Repeat cycle 1 ten times. In cycle 2 complete as many reps of the exercise that you can. No rest between exercises and cycles.

Cycle 1
Regular press-ups: × 7
½ sit-ups: × 7
Diamond press-ups: × 7
Leg levers: × 7
Wide push-ups: × 7
Full sit-ups: × 7
Total press-ups: 210
Total sit-ups: 210

Cycle 2
Press-ups (feet on chair): 5 × 10
Dips (between chairs): 3 × 30

Superset

	Arm haulers	Squats
Sets and Reps	3 × 30	3 × 30

My notes: I had to improvise for today's training session, because I am staying away in a hotel for work and I couldn't get to a gym or any other type of equipment.

YOUR TRAINING SESSION

AM

PM **Training session** PT – Upper body

Time trained

Session time

RPE /10

WORKOUT

Cycle 1
Regular press-ups: ×
½ sit-ups: ×
Diamond press-ups: ×
Leg levers: ×
Wide push-ups: ×
Full sit-ups: ×
Total Press-ups:
Total sit-pps:

Cycle 2
Press-ups (feet on chair): 5 ×
Dips (between chairs): 3 ×

Superset

	Arm haulers	Squats
Sets and Reps	×	×

Your notes:

TRAINING SESSION **WEEK 2** DAY 6

MY TRAINING SESSION

AM Rest

PM Training session Weights – Upper body

Time trained 7.30–8.15 p.m.

Session time 45 minutes

RPE 8/10

WORKOUT
Bench press
1 × 20 warm-up – with just Olympic bar
Set and Rep: 1. 20   2. 10   3. 10   4. 10   5. 10
Weight (kg):   40   60   70   70   70

T-bar row
Set and Rep: 1. 10   2. 10   3. 7   4. 8   5. 10
Weight (kg):   30   40   50   50   50

Military press
Set and Rep: 1. 10   2. 10   3. 10   4. 10   5. 10
Weight (kg):   30   35   35   35   35

My notes: I felt as though I pushed my body hard today. I failed on the last set on each exercise on the 10th rep. I only rested for 1 minute 30 seconds between sets, during which time I would stretch the muscle I worked. No legs due to running tomorrow.

YOUR TRAINING SESSION

AM

PM Training session Weights – Upper body

Time trained

Session time

RPE   /10

WORKOUT
Bench press
1 × 20 warm-up – with just Olympic bar
Set and Rep: 1.   2.   3.   4.   5.
Weight (kg):

T-bar row
Set and Rep: 1.   2.   3.   4.   5.
Weight (kg):

Military press
Set and Rep: 1.   2.   3.   4.   5.
Weight (kg):

Your notes:

TRAINING SESSION **WEEK 2** DAY 7

MY TRAINING SESSION

AM Training session CV – Run

Time trained 10.40–11.05 a.m.

Session time 25 minutes

RPE 8/10

PM Rest

WORKOUT
Run – 3 miles
Actual distance: 3.05 miles
Time: 23.03 minutes
Average Pace: 7.41 m/m

My notes: I ran as fast as I could because I was running late to catch a train to work. Put it this way, I felt slightly nauseous at the end, but I did enjoy it.

YOUR TRAINING SESSION

PM Training session CV – Run

Time trained

Session time

RPE /10

PM

WORKOUT
Run – 3 miles
Actual distance: miles
Time: minutes
Average Pace: m/m

Your notes:

WEEK 2 TESTS

Front view of me at the end of week 2.

Back view of me at the end of week 2.

MY WEEKLY TESTS

Weight (kg):   83
Height (cm):   175.5
BMI: 26.9
RHR: 68
BP: 134/79
Fat %:   16.8

Measurements (cm)
Neck: 38.74
Chest: 101.60
Arm: R 34.92   L 34.92
Navel: 86.36
Hips: 86.36
Thighs: R 60.96   L 60.96
Calves: R 39.37   L 39.37

YOUR WEEKLY TESTS

Weight (kg):
Height (cm):
BMI:
RHR:
BP:
Fat %:

Measurements (cm)
Neck:
Chest:
Arm: R   L
Navel:
Hips:
Thighs: R   L
Calves: R   L

WEEK THREE NUTRITION PLAN WEEK 3

WEEK 3 OVERVIEW

Day	Breakfast	Lunch	Dinner
1	Fruit salad	Chicken wrap	Lemon sole
2	Fruit porridge	Tuna salad with sweet potato	Chicken hot pot
3	Muesli with fresh fruit	Chicken hot pot pitta	Cod and spinach parcels
4	Wheat biscuits or muesli with fruit	Egg salad	Stir fried pork
5	Fresh fruit and seeds	Salmon salad	Chicken yoghurt
6	Omelette	Butternut squash and coriander soup	Lime tuna steaks
7	Fruit smoothie 1	Chicken salad pitta	Beef and sweet potato pie

SHOPPING LIST **WEEK 3**

CARBOHYDRATES
1 bag of brown rice
240g of muesli
10 Charlotte potatoes
10 new potatoes
1 bag of pine nuts
8 wholemeal or brown pitta
  breads
560g porridge oats
1 bag of rice noodles
1 bag of sunflower and
  pumpkin seeds
4 organic tortilla wraps
6 sweet potatoes
Wheat biscuits

DAIRY AND NON-DAIRY ALTERNATIVES
12 eggs
680ml skimmed/soya/rice/
  oat milk
1.7kg soya yoghurt

FISH
200g × 4 cod fillets
4 cooked salmon fillets
4 lemon sole
175g x 4 tuna steaks
4 small tins tuna

MEAT
800g lean minced beef
16 chicken breasts
800g chicken thigh fillets
400g lean ham
450g pork fillets

FRUIT
3 apples
2 apricots

8 bananas
1 lemon
2 limes
3 oranges
2 mangos
1 melon
1 punnet of raspberries

VEGETABLES
2 avocados
115g baby corn
4 baby gem lettuce
600g baby spinach
400g bamboo shoots
175g broccoli
200g button mushrooms
300g cherry tomatoes
2 butternut squash
8 carrots
7 celery sticks
2 courgettes
1 cucumber
3 leeks
3 lettuces
450g mangetout
11 onions
225g frozen peas
1 red onions
4 red peppers
14 red tomatoes
100g rocket salad
13 spring onions
6 yellow peppers

HERBS
Basil
Black pepper
Coriander
Cumin
Dill

Fresh ginger
1 garlic clove
1 lemon thyme sprig
Nutmeg
Parsley
Rosemary
Turmeric

OTHER
Balsamic vinegar
Beef stock
Chicken stock
Chinese rice wine
Cider vinegar
Cold-pressed extra virgin
  olive oil
Corn flour
Dijon mustard
Plain flour
Dark soy sauce
115ml red wine
Soy sauce
400g tinned tomatoes
Vegetable stock
115ml white wine
White wine vinegar

SNACKS
Fruits
Wholegrain crispbread/
  crackers
Crackers/flat breads
Small bowl of muesli
Yoghurt/soya yoghurt
Nuts (cashew, pine or
  occasionally mixed nuts)
Soya nuts
Seeds (pumpkin or sunflower)

FRUIT DRINKS
1 carton fruit juice

RECIPES **WEEK 3** DAY 1

BREAKFAST FRUIT SALAD   *See page 85*

LUNCH CHICKEN WRAP

4 chicken breasts, cooked and cut into strips

4 organic wholewheat tortilla wraps (served hot or cold)

200g mixed salad

4–5 tomatoes, sliced

1 red onion, finely chopped

1 yellow pepper, cut into strips

2 tablespoons of soya/plain yoghurt

1 Heat ½ tablespoon extra virgin olive oil in a frying pan over a medium heat.
2 Cook four chicken breasts for 8–12 minutes or until cooked.
3 Place mixed salad, red onion, yellow pepper, tomatoes and chicken in salad bowl and mix well.
4 Place tortilla wraps on plates, add mixture from salad bowl and roll wrap.
5 Drizzle over soya/plain yoghurt.

DINNER LEMON SOLE

1 small onion, finely chopped

4 lemon sole fillets (175g each)

2 garlic cloves, sliced thinly

4 lemon thyme sprigs

1 lemon, grated rind and juice

2 tablespoons olive oil

Brown rice

Vegetables of your choice (e.g. courgette, spring onion)

1 Preheat oven to 180°C (350°F). Boil the rice and grill the vegetables you have chosen.
2 Place sole fillets in large ovenproof dish and sprinkle onion on top. Add garlic and two lemon thyme sprigs on top of the fillets and season with pepper.
3 Mix lemon juice and olive oil in a small bowl and pour over fish.
4 Bake in oven for 15 minutes or until fish flakes easily.
5 Sprinkle on the lemon rind and the rest of the lemon thyme sprigs and serve with rice and vegetables.

Lunch for tomorrow:
TUNA SALAD WITH SWEET POTATO
Consider preparing sweet potatoes in advance and refrigerate overnight.

RECIPES **WEEK 3** DAY 2

BREAKFAST FRUIT PORRIDGE

See page 81

LUNCH TUNA SALAD
WITH SWEET POTATO

See page 83

DINNER CHICKEN HOT POT

Olive oil, 2 tablespoons

800g chicken thigh fillets, diced

225ml chicken stock

400g tinned chopped tomatoes

115ml white wine

2 cloves garlic, crushed

Corn flour

2 celery sticks, chopped

2 tablespoons rosemary, chopped

2 carrots, finely sliced

2 leeks, washed and sliced

Charlotte potatoes

1 Heat olive oil in large pan over high heat.
2 Add the chicken in batches and cook for 5 minutes or until brown, and remove from pan once cooked.
3 Reduce heat to medium, add the leeks and cook for 8 minutes or until soft.
4 Add the carrots, celery and garlic and cook for a further 10–12 minutes until soft.
5 Add the stock, wine and tomatoes and bring to boil.
6 Reduce heat to low and return chicken with some corn flour (to thicken the sauce) and simmer gently for 35 minutes.
7 Add herbs to taste and serve with Charlotte potatoes.

Lunch for tomorrow:
CHICKEN HOT POT PITTA
Cook four chicken breasts (one per person) for tomorrow's lunch, or use any remaining chicken and sauce from today's hot pot.

RECIPES **WEEK 3** DAY 3

BREAKFAST MUESLI WITH FRESH FRUIT

See page 80

LUNCH CHICKEN HOT POT PITTA

4 chicken breasts, cooked and diced

4 wholemeal pitta breads (served hot or cold)

Sauce from last night's dinner

Lettuce, 4 handfuls washed and chopped

1 red pepper, sliced

1 yellow pepper, sliced

½ red onion, finely sliced

1 Use any remaining chicken and sauce from the hot pot.
2 Heat ½ tablespoon extra virgin olive oil in a frying pan over a medium heat.
3 Cook the chicken for 8–12 minutes or until cooked.
4 Slice open the pitta bread and fill with chicken and salad and pour in the sauce.
5 Serve with salad.

DINNER COD AND SPINACH PARCELS

4 × 200g cod (or barramundi), with skin removed

200g baby spinach leaves

1 tablespoon, ginger

3 spring onions, finely sliced

2 tablespoons soy sauce

Coriander, handful

Lime wedges

Brocoli

Brown rice

1 Preheat oven to 220°C (425°F). Boil the rice and broccoli.
2 Get a large sheet of foil and place half of the spinach leaves in the middle. Add a piece of fish on top then sprinkle with a quarter of ginger, spring onion and drizzle with 2 teaspoons of soy sauce.
3 Wrap the fish in the foil, folding the corners in to ensure the foil is well sealed.
4 Repeat this process with the rest of the fish for each person.
5 Place the four parcels in a baking dish and bake for 15 minutes.
6 Carefully open each parcel and slide contents on to plate.
7 Serve with broccoli and brown rice.

Lunch for tomorrow:
EGG SALAD
Consider preparing eggs in advance (refrigerate overnight).

RECIPES **WEEK 3** DAY 4

BREAKFAST WHEAT BISCUITS OR MUESLI WITH FRUIT

See page 84

LUNCH EGG SALAD

4 baby gem lettuces

200g baby spinach

150g cherry tomatoes, halved

4 shelled hard-boiled eggs, cut into quarters

½ cucumber, sliced

1 yellow pepper, deseeded and sliced

For the dressing:

1 tablespoon Dijon mustard

1 tablespoon olive oil

2 teaspoons cider vinegar

1 teaspoon water

1 Arrange the lettuce, spinach, tomatoes, yellow pepper and cucumber on plates.
2 Mix the mustard and water together, combine with the olive oil and vinegar in a small bowl.
3 Put the eggs on top of the salad, drizzle with the dressing and serve.

DINNER STIR FRIED PORK

450g lean pork fillet, cut into strips

1 tablespoon, olive oil,

16 button mushrooms

115g baby corn

1 garlic clove, finely chopped

Fresh ginger, 2.5cm finely chopped

400g mangetout

400g bamboo shoots, drained and sliced

2 teaspoons dark soy sauce

2 teaspoons Chinese rice wine

225ml vegetable or chicken stock

2 teaspoons corn flour

1 tablespoon water

1 carrot, finely sliced

1–2 spring onions, trimmed and cut lengthways

Rice or rice noodles

For the marinade:

1 tablespoon dark soy sauce

1 tablespoon Chinese rice wine

2 teaspoons corn flour

Pepper

1 Mix the marinade ingredients together in a dish and season with pepper.
2 Add the pork to the marinade, cover and chill for 20 minutes.
3 Blanch the baby corn in boiling water for a few minutes.
4 Drain and refresh in cold water.
5 Heat half the olive oil in a preheated wok and add the pork. Stir fry for 5 minutes until browned. Remove and reserve.
6 Wipe the wok and add the remaining oil and heat. Next, place in the garlic and cook until golden, adding the ginger, mangetout, bamboo shoots and mushrooms and fry for 3 minutes.
7 Stir in the soy sauce, Chinese rice wine, stock and the reserved liquid from pork.
8 Cook for 2–3 minutes then mix the corn flour and water and stir until thickened.
9 Return the pork to the heat stirring in the carrot.
10 Garnish with spring onions and serve with rice or rice noodles.

RECIPES **WEEK 3** DAY 5

BREAKFAST FRESH FRUIT AND SEEDS

See page 82

LUNCH SALMON SALAD

200g mixed salad leaves

¼ cucumber, roughly chopped

4 cooked poach salmon fillets, bite size pieces

2 yellow peppers, sliced

2 tablespoons coriander, chopped

250g cherry tomatoes, halved

For the dressing:

500g soya/plain yoghurt

2 tablespoons coriander, chopped

1 garlic clove, finely chopped

4 teaspoons lemon juice

1 teaspoon cumin, ground

1 For the dressing, place all ingredients in a bowl and mix together; season with black pepper.
2 Cover and refrigerate for 5–10 minutes before using (if the sauce is too thick, add some water to thin out).
3 Arrange salad leaves, cherry tomatoes, spring onions, salmon, cucumber and yellow pepper in a salad bowl and toss.
4 Add salmon on top of salad.
5 Drizzle the dressing over and serve.

DINNER CHICKEN YOGHURT

1 tablespoon plain flour

4 lean chicken breasts, diced skinless

1 tablespoon olive oil

8 small onions, chopped

2 garlic cloves, crushed

225ml chicken stock

2 carrots, chopped

2 celery sticks, chopped

225g frozen peas

1 yellow pepper, sliced and deseeded

115g button mushrooms, sliced

125ml low fat soya/plain yoghurt

3 tablespoons fresh parsley, chopped

10 new potatoes

1 Spread flour over a dish and season with pepper and add chicken. Coat with flour.
2 Heat olive oil in large saucepan and add the onions and garlic and cook over low heat, stirring occasionally for 5 minutes.
3 Add chicken and cook for 10 minutes continuously stirring.
4 Stir in the chicken stock, carrots, peas and celery.
5 Bring to boil and then reduce the heat. Cover and simmer for 5 minutes.
6 Add the peppers and mushrooms, cover and simmer for a further 10 minutes.
7 Stir in the soya/plain yoghurt and chopped parsley and cook for a further 1–2 minutes.
8 Serve with new potatoes.

RECIPES **WEEK 3** DAY 6

BREAKFAST OMELETTE   *See page 88*

LUNCH BUTTERNUT SQUASH AND CORIANDER SOUP   *See page 88*

DINNER LIME TUNA STEAKS

4 × 175g tuna steaks, trim the skin

2 teaspoons, olive oil

½ teaspoon grated lime zest

1 garlic glove, crushed

1 teaspoon ground cumin

1 teaspoon ground coriander

1 tablespoon lime juice

Small handful of fresh coriander, chopped

Salad leaves

For the relish:

2 avocados, peeled and chopped

1 tablespoon lime juice

½ red onion, cut finely

2 tomatoes, chopped

1 Mix the avocados, lime juice, red onion and tomatoes together in a small bowl.
2 To make the paste, mix lime zest, olive oil, garlic, ground cumin and ground coriander in bowl.
3 Spread paste thinly on both sides of the tuna while heating a non-stick pan until hot, and press the tuna steaks into pan to seal them.
4 Reduce heat and cook for 5 minutes. Turn tuna steaks over and cook for a further 4–5 minutes, or until cooked through.
5 Remove tuna from pan and drain on kitchen paper.
6 Transfer fish to plates, serve with salad leaves and relish.
7 Sprinkle 1 tablespoon of lime juice over the top, garnish with fresh coriander.

RECIPES **WEEK 3** DAY 7

BREAKFAST FRUIT SMOOTHIE 1   *See page 87*

LUNCH CHICKEN SALAD PITTA

4 pitta breads, hot or cold

½ tablespoon olive oil

4 lean chicken breasts, sliced into strips

4 tablespoons fresh basil, chopped

1 red pepper

2 spring onions, finely chopped

150g cherry tomatoes, halved

2 tablespoons pine nuts

200g baby spinach

For the dressing:

¼ of a cucumber, finely grated

4 tablespoons soya/plain yoghurt

1 tablespoons olive oil

1 teaspoon balsamic vinegar

2 teaspoons black pepper

2 teaspoons dried dill

1 Pour the olive oil in a frying pan or wok, on a medium heat.
2 Add chicken strips and cook for 8 minutes, or until golden brown. Keep stirring.
3 Add the red pepper, spring onions, tomatoes and pine nuts and cook for a few minutes, while stirring.
4 Place all dressing ingredients in a small bowl and mix well.
5 Slice open the pitta bread and add the chicken, vegetables and spinach. Drizzle over dressing and garnish with basil.

DINNER BEEF AND SWEET POTATO PIE

800g lean minced beef

2 tablespoons olive oil

1 onion, finely chopped

1 leek, finely chopped

1 carrot, finely chopped

1 stick celery, finely chopped

4 tomatoes, diced

2 sweet potatoes, peeled and chopped

1 medium butternut squash, peeled and chopped

2 cloves of garlic, finely chopped

115ml beef stock

1 tablespoon flour

115ml red wine

1 tablespoon rosemary, chopped

Salad leaves

1 Preheat the oven to 180°C (350°F). Heat a large pan of water, boil the sweet potatoes and butternut squash for 10 minutes, or until soft when pierced with knife.

2 Heat a large pan, add olive oil and brown the mince in small batches.

3 Once the mince is cooked, add the onion, leek, carrot, celery and garlic, and cook for 4 minutes.

4 Add stock, flour, wine, tomatoes and rosemary and bring to boil. Simmer for 25 minutes.

5 Mash the sweet potatoes and butternut squash in a bowl.

6 Put mince mixture in large ovenproof dish and place mash on top.

7 Cook for 20 minutes and serve with salad leaves.

Lunch for tomorrow:
BEAN SALAD
Consider preparing eggs in advance (refrigerate overnight).

TRAINING DIARY **WEEK 3**

WEEK 3 OVERVIEW
Day 1: Rest
Day 2: Rest
Day 3: CV – Run
Day 4: Rest
Day 5: Weights – Back and shoulders
Day 6: CV – Run
Day 7: CV – Walk; Weights – Chest
Any day: Myo Stretch

MY DIARY

Day 1 (Monday)
Feeling tired from lack of sleep and I know I need to have an early night tonight. The good side is my hair and skin are looking amazing.
Tiredness 7
Stress 6
Sleep 6 hours 30 minutes

Day 2 (Tuesday)
Worked until a relatively normal time so I had enough time to meet my brother and have a catch up in the pub, then have dinner with him.
Tiredness 5
Stress 5
Sleep 7 hours 30 minutes

Day 3 (Wednesday)
I went for a nice run around Hyde Park and felt amazing afterwards.
Tiredness 5
Stress 5
Sleep 5 hours 40 minutes

Day 4 (Thursday)
My legs were feeling tired after the run, but it is my last day in London before going home. I got back at 10.00 p.m. and then had dinner at 10:15 p.m. with Alison after she finished work.
Tiredness 5
Stress 4
Sleep 7 hours 30 minutes

Day 5 (Friday)
Had a day off work: I had a lie in and went for a walk around Lymington marshes with Alison. Went to the gym and then walked my dog after dinner.
Tiredness 3
Stress 3
Sleep 7 hours 20 minutes

Day 6 (Saturday)
Spent the day with my family and friends, and managed to fit a run in as well.
Tiredness 3
Stress 3
Sleep 7 hours

Day 7 (Sunday)
I'm feeling really good today after the tests, and the pictures are showing some really good progress. Went for another walk and caught the sun for the first time this year. I also trained outside in the back garden.
Tiredness 2
Stress 2
Sleep 6 hours 45 minutes

TRAINING SESSION **WEEK 3** DAY 3

MY TRAINING SESSION

AM Training session CV – Run

Time trained 8.40–9.20 p.m.

Session time 40 minutes

RPE 7/10

PM Rest

WORKOUT
Run – 5 miles
Actual distance: 4.89 miles
Time: 37 minutes
Average Pace: 7.40 m/m

My notes: I ran around Hyde Park and other parks close by. To maximise the distance I ran around the outside edge. Luckily, or unluckily some might say, I found a sand track that was about 1.5 miles long. I ran on that and the grass because it is better for my joints – and it also made it harder.

YOUR TRAINING SESSION

PM Training session CV – Run

Time trained

Session time

RPE /10

PM

WORKOUT
Run – 5 miles
Actual distance: miles
Time: minutes
Average Pace: m/m

Your notes:

TRAINING SESSION **WEEK 3** DAY 5

MY TRAINING SESSION

AM Rest

PM Training session Weights – Back and shoulders

Time trained 6.20–7.20 p.m.

Session time 1 hour

RPE 6/10

WORKOUT

Regular pull-ups
1–10 and 10–1
Total: 110

Bent-over lat raise
Set and Rep:	1. 10	2. 10	3. 10	4. 10
Weight (lb):	17.5	22.5	30	30

Heavy upright rows
Set and Rep:	1. 10	2. 8	3. 6	4. 4
Weight (kg):	30	45	47.5	50

Dumbbell press
Set and Rep:	1. 10	2. 10	3. 10	4. 10	5. 10	6. 10	7. 10
Weight (lb):	7.5	12.5	17.5	22.5	30	40	50

My notes: forced reps – I failed on the 7th set after seven reps, but held the weights for 12 seconds to partially recover then completed three more reps.

It's felt like a long time since I have last been to the gym, due to working away from home. This is a nice session to bring you back into the swing of things. I worked really hard to make sure I made good progress.

YOUR TRAINING SESSION

AM

PM Training session Weights – Back and shoulders

Time trained

Session time

RPE /10

WORKOUT

Regular pull-ups

Total:

Bent-over lat raise
Set and Rep:	1.	2.	3.	4.
Weight (lb):				

Heavy upright rows
Set and Rep:	1.	2.	3.	4.
Weight (kg):				

Dumbbell press
Set and Rep:	1.	2.	3.	4.	5.	6.	7.
Weight (lb):							

Your notes:

TRAINING SESSION **WEEK 3** DAY 6

MY TRAINING SESSION

AM Rest

PM **Training session** CV – Run

Time trained 2.55–3.20 p.m.

Session time 25 minutes

RPE 8/10

WORKOUT
Run – 3 miles
Actual distance: 2.98 miles
Time: 21.26 minutes
Average Pace: 7.08 m/m

My notes: I ran as fast and as hard as possible until I got tired, and this includes running up the hills.

With these three-mile runs, I pushed myself to a point at which I felt completely wiped out, but I listened to my body and when it told me to slow down I then slowed it down.

YOUR TRAINING SESSION

AM

PM **Training session** CV – Run

Time trained

Session time

RPE /10

WORKOUT
Run – 3 miles
Actual distance: miles
Time: minutes
Average Pace: m/m

Your notes:

TRAINING SESSION **WEEK 3** DAY 7

MY TRAINING SESSION

AM Training session CV – Walk

Time trained 9.55–10.55 a.m.

Session time 1 hour

RPE 2/10

PM Training session Weights – Chest

Time trained 4.00–4.50 p.m.

Session time 50 minutes

RPE 6/10

WORKOUT
Walk – 4 miles
Location: Sandbanks to Bournemouth and back.
Incline press
Set and Rep: 1. 10   2. 10   3. 10   4. 10   5. 10
Weight (kg):   40   50   60   70   70
Pec fly
Set and Rep: 1. 10   2. 10   3. 10   4. 10   5. 10
Weight (lb): 30   40   50   52.5   52.5
Morey squeeze (upper)
Set and Rep: 1. 10   2. 10   3. 10   4. 10
Weight (lb): 25   20   20   20
Press-ups (any type)
2, 4, 6, 8, 10
10, 8, 6, 4 and 2
Total: 55

My notes: I just did regular press-ups. I trained outside in my back garden with my friends. All gyms should have these types of facilities. I didn't go too hard in this workout as I was still aching from the last two sessions.

YOUR TRAINING SESSION

AM Training session CV – Walk

Time trained

Session time

RPE   /10

PM Training session Weights – Chest

Time trained

Session time

RPE   /10

WORKOUT
Walk – 4 miles
Location:
Incline press
Set and Rep: 1.   2.   3.   4.   5.
Weight (kg):
Pec fly
Set and Rep: 1.   2.   3.   4.   5.
Weight (lb):
Morey squeeze (upper)
Set and Rep: 1.   2.   3.   4.
Weight (lb):
Press-ups (any type)

Total:

Your notes:

WEEK 3 TESTS

Front view of me at the end of week 3.

Back view of me at the end of week 3.

MY WEEKLY TESTS

Weight (kg):   81.5
Height (cm):   175.5
BMI: 26.5
RHR: 60
BP: 139/69
Fat %:   16

Measurements (cm)
Neck: 38.74
Chest: 102.87
Arm: R 35.56   L 35.56
Navel: 84.45
Hips: 86.36
Thighs: R 60.96   L 60.96
Calves: R 40   L 40

YOUR WEEKLY TESTS

Weight (kg):
Height (cm):
BMI:
RHR:
BP:
Fat %:

Measurements (cm)
Neck:
Chest:
Arm: R   L
Navel:
Hips:
Thighs: R   L
Calves: R   L

WEEK **FOUR** NUTRITION PLAN **WEEK 4**

WEEK 4 OVERVIEW

Day	Breakfast	Lunch	Dinner
1	Fresh fruit and seeds	Bean salad	Mediterranean steaks
2	Wheat biscuits or muesli with fruit	Tuna salad	Stir fried turkey ginger
3	Fruit salad	Beetroot soup	Baked trout
4	Fruit porridge	Chicken wrap	Pork and baked apples
5	Muesli with fresh fruit	Mackerel and potato salad	Tuna pak choi
6	Omelette	Tomato and pepper soup	Ratatouille lamb chops
7	Fruit smoothie 1	Tuna and olive salad	Lemon roasted chicken

SHOPPING LIST **WEEK 4**

CARBOHYDRATES
400g baked potatoes
1 bag of brown rice
810g kidney beans
250g couscous
240g of muesli
400g pinto beans
400g new potatoes
520g porridge oats
1 bag of rice noodles
1 bag of sunflower and
  pumpkin seeds
4 organic tortilla wraps
1 bag of sesame seeds
8 sweet potatoes
Wheat biscuits

DAIRY AND NON-DAIRY ALTERNATIVES
12 eggs
680ml skimmed/soya/rice/
  oat milk
1.7kg soya yoghurt

FISH
8 anchovy fillets
4 × 200g cod fillets
4 cooked mackerel fillets
4 × 2000g tuna steaks
4 small tins tuna
4 whole trout

MEAT
4 chicken breasts
1 large whole chicken
400g lean ham
800g lamb chop
800g pork fillet
4 turkey breasts

FRUIT
12 apples
8 bananas
1 punnet of blueberries
5 lemons
2 limes
2 mangos
1 melon
1 punnet of raspberries
1 punnet of strawberries

VEGETABLES
4 aubergines
2 avocados
8 asparagus
500g raw beetroot
16 × 25g black olives
500g cherry tomatoes
2 carrots
2 celery sticks
4 courgettes
½ cucumber
225g French beans
250g green beans
2 lettuces
50g mangetout
7 onions
3 pak choi
4 parsnips
50g frozen peas
115g plum tomatoes
3 red onions
12 spring onions
7 red peppers
750g red tomatoes
100g rocket salad
200g savoy cabbage
1 turnip
1 yellow pepper

HERBS
Basil
1 Bay leaf
Black pepper
Black peppercorns
Chilli powder
Chives
Cinnamon
Dill
Coriander
Coriander seeds
Cumin
Fresh ginger
Garam masala
1 garlic bulb
Ground fennel
Mint
Oregano
Parsley
Red chilli
Rosemary

OTHER
Balsamic vinegar
Chicken stock
Chinese rice wine
Cold-pressed extra virgin
  olive oil
Corn flour
Dijon mustard
Fish stock
Peanut oil
Red wine vinegar
Sun-dried tomato paste
Soy sauce
Brown sugar
400g tinned tomatoes
Tomato purée
Vegetable stock
White wine vinegar

SNACKS
Fruit
Wholegrain crispbread
  crackers
Flat breads
Small bowl of muesli
Yoghurt/soya yoghurt
Nuts (cashew, pine or
  occasionally mixed nuts)
Soya nuts
Seeds (pumpkin or sunflower)

FRUIT DRINKS
1 carton Fruit juice

RECIPES **WEEK 4** DAY 1

BREAKFAST FRESH FRUIT AND SEEDS

See page 82

LUNCH BEAN SALAD

See page 103

DINNER MEDITERRANEAN STEAKS

4 cod steaks – 140g per steak

150ml fish stock

1 bay leaf

6 black peppercorns

Lemon rind

Lemon wedges

1 small onion, sliced

Parsley

Couscous

For the sauce:

400g chopped tomatoes canned

1 garlic clove, finely chopped

1 tablespoon sun-dried tomato paste

16 black olives (optional)

1 To make the sauce, place the chopped tomatoes, garlic, tomato paste and olives in a large heavy-based saucepan over a low heat. Heat gently, stirring occasionally.

2 Meanwhile, place the fish in a shallow ovenproof casserole dish and pour over the fish stock and add the peppercorns, bay leaf, lemon rind and onion. Bring to the boil, cover and simmer for 10 minutes.

3 Transfer cod to a serving plate and keep warm while water boils for the couscous.

4 Next, sieve the fish stock into the sauce and stir over a medium heat until reduced.

5 Pour the sauce over the fish, garnish with parsley and lemon wedges. Serve with couscous.

Lunch for tomorrow:
TUNA SALAD
Consider preparing sweet potatoes in advance (refrigerate overnight).

RECIPES **WEEK 4** DAY 2

BREAKFAST WHEAT BISCUITS OR MUESLI WITH A FRUIT

See page 84

LUNCH TUNA SALAD

4 cooked sweet potatoes

4 small tinned tuna

1 tablespoon balsamic vinegar

1 tablespoon olive oil

Side salad:

100g of rocket leaves

4 tomatoes, roughly chopped

¼ cucumber, roughly chopped

50g mangetout

1 red pepper, sliced

1 Preheat oven to 190°C (375°F).
2 Cut the sweet potatoes into small chunks, drizzle olive oil over the top and place into the oven for 30–40 minutes.
3 Once cooked, allow to cool and place into the fridge for tomorrow's lunch.
4 Place rocket leaves, mangetout, tomatoes, cucumber and red pepper in a salad bowl and gently mix with balsamic vinegar and olive. Serve with the tuna and sweet potatoes.

DINNER STIR FRIED TURKEY GINGER

2 teaspoons sesame seeds

1 tablespoon sesame oil

800g skinless turkey breasts, cut into thin strips

1 onion, quartered

1 red pepper, deseeded and sliced

2 tablespoons soy sauce

Chinese rice wine, splash of

1 pak choi, halved

1 3cm piece of ginger

1 garlic clove, crushed

1 red chilli, finely sliced

Brown rice

1 Heat a wok/large frying pan over medium heat, add the sesame seeds, stir until lightly toasted and then set aside.
2 Steam pak choi in a steamer for 2–3 minutes, then remove and set aside. Boil water for the rice.
3 Add the turkey to the wok/frying pan and stir fry for 6–8 minutes, or until the turkey is cooked. Remove from wok and set aside. Wipe out wok with paper towel.
4 Return wok to heat and add the rest of the sesame oil with the ginger, garlic, chilli, onion and red pepper, and stir fry for 2 minutes.
5 Return turkey to wok, add rice wine, soy sauce and stir. Add pak choi and stir.
6 Serve with rice and a sprinkle the toasted sesame seeds.

RECIPES **WEEK 4** DAY 3

BREAKFAST FRUIT SALAD   *See page 85*

LUNCH BEETROOT SOUP

2 onions, peeled and roughly chopped

2 large carrot, peeled and roughly chopped

1 large turnip peeled and roughly chopped

2 celery sticks, roughly chopped

500g raw beetroot, peeled and chopped

400g potatoes, washed and chopped

200g savoy cabbage

3 garlic cloves, finely sliced

2 litres of vegetable stock

410g tin kidney beans

1 tablespoon red wine vinegar

150g soya/plain yoghurt

1 Put onions, carrots, turnips, celery, beetroot, garlic and vegetable stock in large pan.
2 Bring to the boil and simmer for 30 minutes.
3 Add the potatoes, cabbage, beans and simmer for a further 20–30 minutes or until potatoes are tender.
4 Stir in the vinegar and the yoghurt.
5 Serve soup in bowls.

DINNER BAKED TROUT

4 sweet potatoes, roughly chopped

1 courgette, roughly chopped

2 red peppers, roughly chopped

250g cherry tomatoes

1 medium red onion, roughly chopped

4 fresh trout, gutted

Black pepper

2 teaspoons coriander

1 teaspoon cinnamon

2 teaspoons oregano

2 teaspoons basil

1 clove garlic, finely chopped

1 tablespoon olive oil

1 Preheat the oven to 190°C (375°F).
2 Pre-boil the sweet potatoes in saucepan of water, until potatoes are slightly soft. Drain water.
3 Place the sweet potatoes, courgette, tomatoes red pepper, all the herbs, garlic and onion in a baking dish and drizzle over the olive oil.
4 Bake for 10–15 minutes, or until the vegetables are cooked, stirring vegetables occasionally.
5 Meanwhile, preheat grill to medium/high and place the fish on grill tray.
6 Drizzle over a little olive oil and season with black pepper and cook for 5–6 minutes each side, or until fish is cooked.
7 Arrange vegetables on serving plate and place fish on top.

RECIPES **WEEK 4** DAY 4

BREAKFAST FRUIT PORRIDGE

See page 81

LUNCH CHICKEN WRAP

See page 113

DINNER PORK AND BAKED APPLES

1 × 800g lean pork fillet, remove fat

2 tablespoon ground fennel

2 tablespoons olive oil

2 apples, cored and quartered

2 teaspoons brown sugar

2 tablespoons water

4 parsnips, peeled and chopped into chunks

Rosemary, 4 sprigs

200g green beans

1 Preheat oven to 180°C (350°F).
2 Season the pork with pepper and roll in the fennel.
3 Wrap in cling film and refrigerate for 10–15 minutes.
4 Heat a large frying pan over a high heat and cook the pork with half the olive oil on each side for 3 minutes, or until golden. Set aside and cover.
5 Place apples in an ovenproof dish, sprinkle the brown sugar and water. Cover with foil and set aside.
6 Place parsnip, rosemary and remaining oil in a baking dish and toss to coat. Bake for 10 minutes.
7 Place apples into the oven, and at the same time add the pork to the parsnip dish. After a further 10 minutes of cooking the parsnips should be golden, the pork cooked and the apples soft.
8 Meanwhile, bring a small saucepan of water to the boil and add the beans. Cook for 5 minutes.
9 Serve immediately.

Lunch for tomorrow:
MACKEREL AND POTATO SALAD
Consider preparing potatoes in advance (refrigerate overnight).

RECIPES **WEEK 4** DAY 5

BREAKFAST MUESLI WITH FRESH FRUIT

See page 80

LUNCH MACKEREL AND POTATO SALAD

4 mackerel fillets (250g each)

4 teaspoons Dijon mustard

Serve with green beans

For the potato salad:

400g new potatoes

4 spring onions, roughly chopped

1 tablespoon fresh dill, chopped

1 tablespoon chives, chopped

1 tablespoon parsley, chopped

1. Steam the potatoes for 20 minutes or until tender.
2. Mix the spring onions, dill, chives, parsley, lemon juice, potatoes and fromage frais in a salad bowl.
3. Preheat the grill to high and wash the mackerel. Pat dry with kitchen towel, making sure the black skin from the gut has been removed.
4. Lay the fillets skin-side down and spread the mustard on the flesh.
5. Grill the mackerel for 5 minutes until the flesh is no longer translucent.
6. Serve with potato salad and green beans.

DINNER TUNA PAK CHOI

4 × 200g tuna steaks

2 teaspoons peanut oil

2 pak choi, leaves separated and washed

4 spring onions, finely sliced

1 tablespoon fresh coriander

1 tablespoon mint leaves

Lime wedges

For the dressing:

2 tablespoon light soy sauce

2 teaspoons lime juice

1 teaspoon ginger, grated

1. In a small bowl mix all the dressing ingredients.
2. Heat frying pan over medium heat and brush tuna steaks with peanut oil.
3. Add tuna to pan and cook for 4 minutes on each side.
4. Use a steamer to cook pak choi for 2–3 minutes.
5. Arrange the pak choi on a serving plate and place tuna on top.
6. Sprinkle with spring onion, coriander and mint, and drizzle the dressing on top.
7. Use lime wedges to garnish and serve.

RECIPES **WEEK 4** DAY 6

BREAKFAST OMELETTE   *See page 88*

LUNCH TOMATO AND PEPPER SOUP

2 red peppers, deseeded and halved

2 tablespoons olive oil

1 large onion, finely sliced

2 cloves of garlic, crushed

1 tablespoon tomato paste

750g tomatoes, roughly chopped

450ml vegetable stock

Basil, handful

1. Preheat oven to 180°C (350°F).
2. Place red peppers in baking tray, skin-side up and drizzle with half the olive oil.
3. Roast for 25 minutes, or until soft and remove from oven. Allow to cool slightly, then roughly chop.
4. Heat the rest of the oil in a large saucepan, over a medium heat.
5. Add the onion and cook until soft.
6. Add garlic and tomato paste and cook for 2 minutes, stirring continuously.
7. Add red pepper, tomato and stock, cover and simmer for 15 minutes.
8. Allow the soup to cool slightly, and gently stir. Season with basil and serve.

DINNER RATATOUILLE LAMB CHOPS

8 lean lamb chops, diced

1 tablespoon olive oil

250g couscous

1 tablespoon ground pepper

2 teaspoons coriander seeds

1 teaspoon garam masala

1 teaspoon chilli powder

For the ratatouille:

2 teaspoons olive oil

4 baby aubergines

1 onion, finely chopped

1 red pepper, deseeded and sliced

1 courgette, sliced

115ml chicken stock

2 tomatoes, sliced

1 tablespoon parsley, chopped

1 clove garlic, finely chopped

1. Mix all the spices in a bowl and brush the chops with a little olive oil. Coat chops with spice mixture, cover with cling film and refrigerate for 1 hour.
2. To make ratatouille, heat the olive oil in a large frying pan over medium heat. Add aubergines and cook for 4 minutes or until golden.
3. Add onion and garlic and cook until lightly coloured. Next add the red pepper and courgette and cook for further minute.
4. Add chicken stock and tomatoes and bring to boil, cook for a further 5 minutes and add parsley and season to taste.
5. Bring water to a boil and add the couscous, cover with a lid and allow to settle.
6. Heat oil in a frying pan over high heat and cook lamb for 3 minutes each side.
7. Serve the lamb chops with ratatouille and couscous.

RECIPES **WEEK 4** DAY 7

BREAKFAST FRUIT SMOOTHIE 1   *See page 87*

LUNCH TUNA AND OLIVE SALAD   *See page 81*

DINNER LEMON ROASTED CHICKEN

4 lemons, 2 × grated zest, 2 × cut into quarters

1 large chicken

1 onion, roughly chopped

50g peas (fresh or frozen)

50g French beans, trimmed

1 courgette, sliced

6–8 asparagus heads, trimmed

600ml chicken stock

Fresh basil, 1 handful chopped

Brown rice

1 Preheat oven to 180°C (350°F). Rub the lemon rind on the chicken and place in a casserole dish.
2 Squeeze lemon juice all over the chicken. Add the vegetables and basil around the chicken.
3 Pour over the stock and put the chicken in oven and cook for 1½ hours.
4 Serve with brown rice.

Lunch for tomorrow:
YELLOW SPLIT PEA SOUP
Soak the yellow split peas overnight for tomorrow's lunch.

TRAINING DIARY **WEEK 4**

WEEK 4 OVERVIEW
Day 1: Rest
Day 2: PT – Upper body; CV – Hill sprints
Day 3: Weights – Back and shoulders
Day 4: CV – Walk; CV – Run
Day 5: Weights – Chest and arms
Day 6: Rest
Day 7: Test day
Any day: Myo stretch

MY DIARY

Day 1 (Monday)
Back up to London for work. I actually walked away feeling ... I believe the word is outstanding.
Tiredness 4
Stress 4
Sleep 7 hours

Day 2 (Tuesday)
I had a broken night's sleep so I didn't felt like going outside to train. I ended up training in the hotel. My upper body was still aching slightly, but that wasn't enough to stop me training.
Tiredness 6
Stress 4
Sleep 8 hours

Day 3 (Wednesday)
I came back from London in the afternoon and once I was back I trained as normal. This meant I didn't eat dinner until 9.50 p.m.
Tiredness 5
Stress 4
Sleep 6 hours 45 minutes

Day 4 (Thursday)
I walked along the seaside with Alison for three miles before going off to work. Later I had a lymphatic massage to help get rid of all my waste and toxins from within my body, and then I went for the three-mile run.
Tiredness 4
Stress 4
Sleep 5 hours

Day 5 (Friday)
By the time I finished work I was feeling a little tired, but during the day I was full of beans.
Tiredness 3
Stress 3
Sleep 7 hours

Day 6 (Saturday)
I had dinner with my parents today, to catch up with them.
Tiredness 3
Stress 3
Sleep 6 hours 50 minutes

Day 7 (Sunday)
Test day today. I was really happy with my progress and results apart from my 1 rep max with the military press. When I finished the tests I had the rest of the day off.
Tiredness 4
Stress 4
Sleep 5 hours 30 minutes

TRAINING SESSION **WEEK 4** DAY 2

MY TRAINING SESSION

AM Rest

PM **Training session** PT – Upper body;
CV – Hill sprints

Time trained 7.15–8.00 p.m.

Session time 45 minutes

RPE 9/10

WORKOUT
Chest and abs cycle × 15
Regular press-ups × 10
Half sit-ups × 7
Diamond press-ups × 10
Leg levers × 7
Wide push-ups × 10
Crunches × 7
Total press-ups: 450
Total sit-ups: 315

Hill sprints or step training
10 × hill sprints/sprint up staircase
I was meant to do hill sprints today, but due to me being away in London I chose to run up the hotel's staircase instead. There were 71 steps in total.

1. 21.03 seconds
2. 20.30 seconds
3. 20.62 seconds
4. 20.59 seconds
5. 20.60 seconds
6. 20.55 seconds
7. 20.62 seconds
8. 17.24 seconds
9. 16.96 seconds
10. 16.92 seconds

My notes: I raced against my first time of 21.03 seconds and then had to beat it for the next nine times. If I failed to beat my original time I would give myself a forfeit. I found the sprinting really hard, as I gave more than I could for each hill. Good luck with this and just keep going.

YOUR TRAINING SESSION

AM

PM **Training session** PT – Upper body;
CV – Hill sprints

Time trained

Session time

RPE   /10

WORKOUT
Chest and abs cycle × 15
Regular press-ups   ×
Half sit-ups   ×
Diamond press-ups   ×
Leg levers   ×
Wide push-ups   ×
Crunches   ×
Total press-ups:
Total sit-ups:

Hill sprints or step training
Sprint with 100 per cent effort up the stairs and then take it easy on the way back down, (approximately 50 per cent effort). If you are running up a hill, you should choose one that takes no longer than 45 seconds to get to the top.

1.   seconds
2.   seconds
3.   seconds
4.   seconds
5.   seconds
6.   seconds
7.   seconds
8.   seconds
9.   seconds
10.   seconds

Your notes:

TRAINING SESSION **WEEK 4** DAY 3

MY TRAINING SESSION

AM Rest

PM Training session Weights – Back and shoulders

Time trained 6.00–7.00 p.m.

Session time 1 hour

RPE 8/10

WORKOUT
Pull-ups
Regular: 2, 4, 6, 8
Close: 2, 4, 6, 8
Wide: 2, 4, 6, 8
Reverse: 2, 4, 6, 8
Mountain climber: 2, 4, 6, 8
Total pull-ups: 100

Military press
1 × 20 warm-up – with just Olympic bar
Set and Rep: 1. 15   2. 10   3. 10   4. 10
Weight (kg):   30   40   45   50

Dumbbell press
Set and Rep: 1. 0   2. 8   3. 10   4. 10
Weight (lb):   30   40   50   55

Bent-over lat raise
Set and Rep: 1. 15   2. 15   3. 10   4. 10
Weight (lb):   17.5   22.5   30   30

My notes: I love the pull-ups. Very hard, but what a session.

YOUR TRAINING SESSION

AM

PM Training session Weights – Back and shoulders

Time trained

Session time

RPE   /10

WORKOUT
Pull-ups
Regular:
Close:
Wide:
Reverse:
Mountain climber:
Total pull-ups:

Military press
1 × 20 warm-up – with just Olympic bar
Set and Rep: 1.   2.   3.   4.
Weight (lb):

Dumbbell press
Set and Rep: 1.   2.   3.   4.
Weight (lb):

Bent-over lat raise
Set and Rep: 1.   2.   3.   4.
Weight (lb):

Your notes:

TRAINING SESSION **WEEK 4** DAY 4

MY TRAINING SESSION

AM Training session CV – Walk

Time trained 8.00–8.45 a.m.

Session time 45 minutes

RPE 2/10

PM Training session CV – Run

Time trained 7.50–8.15 p.m.

Session time 25 minutes

RPE 9/10

WORKOUT
Walk – 3 miles
Run – 3 miles
Actual distance: 3.05 miles
Time: 23.41 minutes
Average Pace: 7.53 m/m

My notes: I went all out for this run, but I ended up burning out after 2.7 miles. It put a bit of a downer on me because it was looking as though I was going to beat my personal best. Instead I got a stitch and felt slightly sick. I was also running against a strong wind until the half-way point, then when I turned around the wind was with me on the way back.

YOUR TRAINING SESSION

AM Training session CV – Walk

Time trained

Session time

RPE   /10

PM Training session CV – Run

Time trained

Session time

RPE   /10

WORKOUT
Walk – 3 miles
Run – 3 miles
Actual distance: miles
Time: minutes
Average Pace: m/m

Your notes:

TRAINING SESSION **WEEK 4** DAY 5

MY TRAINING SESSION

AM Rest

PM **Training session** Weights – Chest and arms

Time trained 5.05–6.35 p.m.

Session time 1 hour 30 minutes

RPE 5/10

WORKOUT
Incline press
1 × 20 warm-up – with just Olympic bar
Set and Rep: 1. 20   2. 10   3. 10   4. 9   5. 7
Weight (kg):   40   50   70   75   75

Bench press
Set and Rep: 1. 10   2. 9   3. 7   4. 8
Weight (kg):   60   90   90   90

Decline press
Set and Rep: 1. 9   2. 9   3. 8
Weight (kg):   90   90   90

Superset
Incline dumbbell curls
Sets and Reps 1. 10   2. 10   3. 10   4. 10
Weight (lb)   50   50   50   50
Supernated curl
Sets and Reps 1. 10   2. 10   3. 10   4. 10
Weight (lb)   7.5   7.5   7.5   7.5

Rope triceps press-downs
30-second rest between sets.
Set and Rep: 1. 20 2. 13 3. 7 4. 8 5. 6 6. 10 7. 10
Weight (kg):   15   15   15   15   15   15   15

YOUR TRAINING SESSION

AM

PM **Training session** Weights – Chest and arms

Time trained

Session time

RPE   /10

WORKOUT
Incline press
1 × 20 warm-up – with just Olympic bar
Set and Rep: 1.   2.   3.   4.   5.
Weight (kg):

Bench press
Set and Rep: 1.   2.   3.   4.
Weight (kg):

Decline press
Set and Rep: 1.   2.   3.
Weight (kg):

Superset
Incline dumbbell curls
Set and Reps: 1.   2.   3.   4.
Weight (lb):
Supernated curl
Set and Reps: 1.   2.   3.   4.
Weight (lb):

Rope triceps press-downs
30-second rest between sets.
Set and Rep: 1.   2.   3.   4.   5.   6.   7.
Weight (kg):

Morey squeeze (upper – cable)
Set and Rep: 1. 10   2. 10   3. 10
Weight (kg):   7.5   7.5   7.5

My notes: I felt so pumped after this workout, it's a really amazing feeling.

Morey squeeze (upper – cable)
Set and Rep: 1.   2.   3.
Weight (kg):

Your notes:

Front view of me at the end of week 4.

Back view of me at the end of week 4.

WEEK 4 HEALTH CHECK

MY RESULTS

Statistics	Weight (kg): 80
	Height (cm): 175.5
Health tests	BMI: 26
	RHR: 57
	BP: 140/58
	Fat (%): 15.1
	Glucose: 5.7
	Cholesterol: 4.6
	Lung function: 640
Measurements (cm)	Neck: 38.73
	Chest: 104.14
	Arms: R: 36.83 L: 36.83
	Navel: 83.18
	Hips: 86.36
	Thighs: R: 60.96 L: 60.96
	Calves: R: 40 L: 40
Calliper test (mm)	Biceps: 3
	Triceps: 7
	Waist: 10
	Subscapularis: 11
	Total: 31
	Calliper fat (%): 13.1
Fitness tests	Bleep test (level): 12.3
Maximum reps in one minute	Push-ups: 59
	½ sit-ups: 60
	Squats: 52
	Dips: 55
	Max pull-ups: 12
One rep maximum weight training (kg)	Squats: 110
	Bench press: 100
	Military press: 60
	Deadlifts: 120

YOUR RESULTS

Statistics	Weight (kg):
	Height (cm):
Health tests	BMI:
	RHR:
	BP: /
	Fat (%):
	Glucose:
	Cholesterol:
	Lung function:
Measurements (cm)	Neck:
	Chest:
	Arms: R: L:
	Navel:
	Hips:
	Thighs: R: L:
	Calves: R: L:
Calliper test (mm)	Biceps:
	Triceps:
	Waist:
	Subscapularis:
	Total:
	Calliper fat (%):
Fitness tests	Bleep test (level):
Maximum reps in one minute	Push-ups:
	½ sit-ups:
	Squats:
	Dips:
	Max pull-ups:
One rep maximum weight training (kg)	Squats:
	Bench press:
	Military press:
	Deadlifts:

WEEK **FIVE** NUTRITION PLAN **WEEK 5**

WEEK 5 OVERVIEW

Day	Breakfast	Lunch	Dinner
1	Fresh fruit and seeds	Yellow split pea soup	Prawn stir fry
2	Wheat biscuits or muesli with fruit	Tuna salad	Lamb stew
3	Muesli with fresh fruit	Lamb pitta	Chicken with lemongrass
4	Fruit porridge	Salmon salad	Fillet of beef
5	Fresh fruit and seeds	Chicken wrap	Barramundi curry
6	Omelette	Beef and beetroot salad	Paella
7	Fruit smoothie 2	Vegetable soup	Roasted chicken

SHOPPING LIST **WEEK 5**

CARBOHYDRATES
6 baking potatoes
1 bag of brown rice
260g of muesli
12 new potatoes
480g porridge oats
225g yellow split peas
200g short grain rice
1 bag of rice noodles
1 bag of sunflower and
  pumpkin seeds
4 organic tortilla wraps
5 sweet potatoes
Wheat biscuits

DAIRY AND NON-DAIRY ALTERNATIVES
8 eggs
150g Greek yoghurt
50g parmesan cheese/goat's
  cheese
1760ml skimmed/soya/rice/
  oat milk
2.5kg soya yoghurt

FISH
800g barramundi fillets
150g calamari
200g mussels
600g raw prawns
4 poached salmon fillets
4 small tins tuna
400g white fish of your choice

MEAT
800g beef fillet
400g cooked roast beef
800g chicken on the bone
4 chicken breasts
1 large whole chicken
400g lean ham
600g boneless lamb

FRUIT

7 apples
2 apricots
9 bananas
1 punnet of blueberries
1 bag of green grapes
3 lemons
1 lime
2 peaches
1 punnet of raspberries

VEGETABLES
16 asparagus
4 cooked beetroot
125g frozen broad beans
250g broccoli
250g cherry tomatoes
7 carrots
4 celery sticks
1 courgette
½ cucumber
3 lettuce
250g mangetout
175g mushrooms
8 onions
275g frozen peas
200g runner beans
1 red onion
1 green pepper
2 red peppers
12 red tomatoes
150g rocket salad
150g baby spinach
21 spring onions
150g sugar snap peas
1 yellow pepper

HERBS

Basil
3 bay leaves
Black pepper
Coriander
Cumin
6 dill sprigs
1 fennel bulb
1 garlic bulb
Fresh ginger
11 lemongrass stalks
Mint
Oregano
Paprika
Parsley
6 peppercorns
Red chilli
Rosemary
Saffron
Thyme

OTHER
Balsamic vinegar
Chicken stock
Chinese white wine vinegar
Cold-pressed extra virgin
  olive oil
Corn flour
Dijon mustard
Fish sauce
Prawn paste
Soy sauce
Brown sugar
800g tinned tomatoes
Tomato purée
Vegetable stock
115ml white wine
Worcestershire sauce

SNACKS
Fruits
Wholegrain crispbread
  crackers
Flat breads
Small bowl of muesli
Yoghurt/soya yoghurt
Nuts (cashew, pine or
  occasionally mixed nuts)
Soya nuts

FRUIT DRINKS
1 carton fruit juice

RECIPES **WEEK 5** DAY 1

BREAKFAST FRESH FRUIT AND SEEDS

See page 82

LUNCH YELLOW SPLIT PEA SOUP

225g yellow split peas (pre-soak for 12 hours overnight in cold water)

1.5 litres of vegetable stock

1 onion, peeled and sliced

1 sweet potato, peeled and chopped

3 carrots, trimmed, peeled and sliced

Fresh mint, handful

Baby spinach leaves, 4 handfuls

1 Drain the water from the split peas.
2 Boil the vegetable stock in a large saucepan, add split peas, then simmer for 25 minutes, removing any scum that appears.
3 Add all the other vegetables and simmer for a further 15–20 minutes, or until vegetables are tender.
4 Remove from heat and allow to cool.
5 Blend soup with food processor or blender.
6 Serve with fresh mint.

DINNER PRAWN STIR FRY

8 spring onions, finely chopped

1 green pepper, finely chopped

1 red pepper, finely chopped

2 tablespoons olive oil

2 garlic cloves, finely chopped

1 tablespoon ginger, finely cut

200g mangetout

450g raw prawns, thawed and peeled

4 tablespoons Chinese rice wine

Rice noodles

1 Heat the olive oil in a big frying pan or wok over a medium to high heat.
2 Add the spring onions, garlic, ginger and peppers to pan and stir fry for 4 minutes, stirring continuously.
3 Add the mangetout and prawns and stir fry for 4 minutes or until prawns have change colour.
4 Stir in rice wine.
5 Serve with rice noodles.

Lunch for tomorrow:
TUNA SALAD
Consider preparing sweet potatoes in advance (refrigerate overnight).

RECIPES **WEEK 5** DAY 2

BREAKFAST WHEAT BISCUITS OR
MUESLI WITH FRUIT

See page 84

LUNCH TUNA SALAD

See page 131

DINNER LAMB STEW

600g lean boneless lamb,
diced into 2.5cm cubes

1 onion, chopped

6 peppercorns

1 fennel bulb

115g mushrooms

1 teaspoon corn flour

1 tablespoon soya milk

150ml soya/plain yoghurt

6 baking potatoes

6 fresh dill sprigs

1 bay leaf

Half a lemon, grated rind and juice

1 Place lamb in large saucepan and cover with cold water.
2 Bring to boil over medium heat, remove any scum that rises to the surface.
3 Add the onion, two dill sprigs, bay leaf and peppercorns. Reduce heat, cover and simmer for 45 minutes.
4 Add the fennel, potatoes and mushrooms and simmer for a further 30 minutes, or until lamb is tender.
5 Using a slotted spoon, transfer the lamb, onion, fennel and mushrooms to a dish and keep warm.
6 Sieve the cooking liquid and reserve 300ml. Pour the reserved cooking liquid into a pan and bring to boil. Mix the corn flour and milk until smooth, then add to the cooking liquid.
7 Reduce the heat and simmer for 5 minutes, keep stirring until thickened.
8 Add the lemon rind and juice to the sauce.
9 Return the lamb, onion, fennel and mushrooms to the sauce pan and simmer for 5 minutes.
10 Meanwhile, mix the yoghurt, and four fresh dill sprigs in a small bowl, then add to the stew.
11 Serve with the potatoes.

Lunch for tomorrow:
LAMB PITTA
Leave some of the lamb and sauce for lunch tomorrow.

RECIPES **WEEK 5** DAY 3

BREAKFAST MUESLI WITH FRESH FRUIT

See page 80

LUNCH LAMB PITTA

4 pitta breads (1 per person)

Use some of last night's dinner including sauce

Rocket leaves, handful per person

4 tomatoes, sliced

1 Slice open the pitta bread
2 Place last night's dinner into the pitta bread with the rocket leaves and sliced tomatoes.

DINNER CHICKEN WITH LEMONGRASS

800g lean chicken pieces on the bone

150g sugar snap peas

16 asparagus

4 spring onions, finely sliced

Lime wedges

Brown rice

For the marinade:

1 lemongrass stalk, finely chopped

2 cloves garlic, crushed

2 teaspoons ginger, grated

2 tablespoons soy sauce

115ml chicken stock

2 teaspoons olive oil

2 tablespoons Chinese rice wine

1 Mix all the marinade ingredients in a bowl.
2 Coat the chicken thoroughly with the marinade.
3 Cover with cling film and refrigerate for up to 2 hours or overnight and, if possible, turn occasionally.
4 Preheat oven 180°C (350°F).
5 Place chicken and marinade into dish and cook for 30 minutes, turning occasionally.
6 Bring a small saucepan of water to the boil and cook asparagus and sugar snap peas for 2–3 minutes.
7 Drain and serve meat, juices and vegetables.

RECIPES **WEEK 5** DAY 4

BREAKFAST FRUIT PORRIDGE

See page 81

LUNCH SALMON SALAD

See page 118

DINNER FILLET OF BEEF

800g beef fillet
3 onions, finely sliced
2 teaspoons olive oil
2 teaspoons balsamic vinegar
8 mushrooms, peeled and stems removed
115ml white wine
100g fresh mixed salad leaves

1 Preheat oven to 180°C (350°F).
2 Cook the onions in olive oil over a medium heat for 20–25 minutes, or until soft. Add the balsamic vinegar and cook for a further 5 minutes.
3 Heat a non-stick frying pan over high heat. Sear fillet on both sides and transfer beef to a baking dish.
4 Place mushrooms on second baking tray, pour over the wine and cover with foil.
5 Place both dishes in the oven and cook for 15 minutes.
6 Remove the beef from oven, cover with foil and leave to rest for 10 minutes.
7 At the same time, remove the foil from the mushrooms and bake for a further 10 minutes.
8 Divide the meat into four portions, serve with mixed salad leaves, caramelised onions and mushrooms.

Lunch for tomorrow:
CHICKEN WRAP
Consider preparing chicken in advance (refrigerate overnight).

RECIPES **WEEK 5** DAY 5

BREAKFAST FRESH FRUIT AND SEEDS

See page 82

LUNCH CHICKEN WRAP

See page 113

DINNER BARRAMUNDI CURRY

1 tablespoon olive oil

800g barramundi fillet, diced

1 teaspoon brown sugar

115ml chicken stock

1 tablespoon fish sauce

200g runner beans

Handful of coriander

Rice or vegetables

For the curry paste:

1 red chilli, roughly chopped

1 lemongrass stalk, finely chopped

2 spring onions, finely chopped

1 clove garlic, roughly chopped

2 teaspoons finely grated ginger

2 teaspoons coriander

1 teaspoon of prawn paste

1 Place all curry paste ingredients in food processor and blend to a fine paste.
2 Boil the rice, or grill the vegetables under a medium heat.
3 Heat olive oil in large non-stick frying pan over a medium heat.
4 Add the curry paste and fish and stir fry for 3 minutes, turning fish carefully to coat with paste.
5 Add the sugar, chicken stock, fish sauce and beans.
6 Cook for a further 5 minutes. Serve with rice/ vegetables.

RECIPES **WEEK 5** DAY 6

BREAKFAST OMELETTE

See page 88

LUNCH BEEF AND BEETROOT SALAD

4 cooked beetroots

50g Parmesan, shaved

400g lean finely sliced cold roast beef

Generous amount of salad and baby spinach

Basil, small handful, chopped

For the dressing:

1 tablespoon balsamic vinegar

2 tablespoons olive oil, cold pressed

1 clove of garlic, chopped

1 teaspoon Dijon mustard

1 Add all dressing ingredients into bowl and whisk well.
2 Add the remaining ingredients into large salad bowl and mix together
3 Pour dressing over the top.

DINNER PAELLA

1 onion, finely chopped

3 tomatoes, roughly chopped

200g short grain rice

1 litre chicken stock

400g fish of your choice

150g uncooked prawns, peeled

200g mussels, bearded and washed

150g calamari

150g peas

Spices and herbs:

1 teaspoon saffron

1 teaspoon paprika

2 cloves of garlic, crushed

Small handful of parsley, roughly chopped

Ground black pepper

Lemon wedges

1 In a small non-stick frying pan, lightly toss saffron and transfer to a cup.
2 Crush and add paprika and 60ml boiling water. Stir to dissolve and set aside.
3 Heat olive oil in large pan over medium heat.
4 Add garlic and onion, and cook for 5 minutes, or until soft.
5 Add the tomatoes and cook for a further 3minutes.
6 Add rice and cook for 5 minutes, stirring continuously. Meanwhile bring the stock to a boil in a large saucepan.
7 Add the stock and saffron liquid to the rice mixture, stir well and simmer for 15 minutes.
8 Add fish, prawns, mussels and calamari on top of rice, cover with foil and cook for10 minutes.
9 Add peas, re-cover pan and cook for a further 5 minutes.
10 Sprinkle with parsley, season with pepper and serve with lemon wedges.

RECIPES **WEEK 5** DAY 7

BREAKFAST FRUIT SMOOTHIE 2

4 tablespoons of nut and seed muesli

1200ml milk (soya/rice/oat or skimmed milk)

2 bananas

2 apricots

2 peaches

1 Mix the muesli and milk in a blender until nearly smooth.
2 Add the bananas, peaches and apricots and blend until completely smooth.
3 If the smoothie is too thick, add more water.

LUNCH TUNA AND OLIVE SALAD

See page 81

DINNER ROASTED CHICKEN

1 tablespoon olive oil

1.5kg lean chicken

1 onion, peeled and roughly chopped

2 cloves of garlic, finely chopped

2 celery stalks, cut into chunks

2 large carrots, cut into chunks

12 new potatoes

1 tablespoon fresh thyme

2 bay leaves

400g tinned chopped tomatoes

1 tablespoon Worcestershire sauce

300ml chicken stock

125g frozen broad beans

125g frozen peas

250g broccoli florets

Freshly ground black pepper

1 Preheat oven to 190°C (375°F).
2 Heat the olive oil in an oven-proof dish, remove any excess fat and set the chicken breast side up in the dish.
3 Add the onion, garlic, celery, carrots, potatoes, thyme and bay leaves.
4 Pour in chopped tomatoes, Worcestershire sauce and stock. Mix together and bring to a simmer.
5 Cover and cook for 1 hour or until chicken is cooked.
6 Carefully remove chicken from casserole dish.
7 Add the frozen peas, broad beans and broccoli, season with pepper and cook for 10 minutes.
8 Carve and serve vegetables with tomato sauce.

Lunch for tomorrow:
CHICKEN SALAD
Keep enough chicken left over for tomorrow's lunch.

TRAINING DIARY **WEEK 5**

WEEK 5 OVERVIEW
Day 1: Rest
Day 2: Weights – Chest and back
Day 3: CV – Run
Day 4: CV – Run PT
Day 5: CV – Walk; CV – Cycle PT
Day 6: Weights – Legs
Day 7: Rest
Any day: Myo stretch

MY DIARY
Day 1 (Monday)
I worked away from home again today. Felt really strong today so I went all out with my exercises.
Tiredness 4
Stress 3
Sleep 6 hours 30 minutes

Day 2 (Tuesday)
Had a sore throat today, but I felt strong in the gym so there wasn't anything wrong with me.
Tiredness 4
Stress 4
Sleep 7 hours

Day 3 (Wednesday)
Had my dog with me all day today. I took her with me for the run, but she got really knackered so I finished it a bit early.
Tiredness 7
Stress 4
Sleep 6 hours 45 minutes

Day 4 (Thursday)
Had an outbreak on my forehead but it wasn't anything major. I'll have to keep my eye on this. My shaving rash has now gone down. I also had a myo massage to keep my body and posture on track.
Tiredness 4
Stress 4
Sleep 7 hours 30 minutes

Day 5 (Friday)
Went for a two-hour walk with Alison and dog, then later I trained outside.
Tiredness 3
Stress 3
Sleep 7 hours

Day 6 (Saturday)
I went shopping with my mum today. Had a really good talk, but got a little stressed with some personal circumstances.
Tiredness 4
Stress 5
Sleep 7 hours 40 minutes

Day 7 (Sunday)
I went to a theme park today to celebrate a birthday.
Tiredness 2
Stress 3
Sleep 6 hours 50 minutes

TRAINING SESSION **WEEK 5** DAY 2

MY TRAINING SESSION

AM Rest

PM Training session Weights – Chest and back

Time trained 6.00–7.00 p.m.

Session time 1 hour

RPE 7/10

WORKOUT

Deadlift
1 × 20 warm-up – with just Olympic bar

Set and Rep:	1. 10	2. 10	3. 10	4. 10	5. 10
Weight (kg):	50	90	100	110	110

Bench press

Set and Rep:	1. 15	2. 10	3. 10	4. 8	5. 7
Weight (kg):	40	60	80	90	100

Superset

	Pull-ups (regular)					Low pull				
Sets	1.	2.	3.	4.	5.	1.	2.	3.	4.	5.
Reps	12	10	8	6	4	10	10	10	10	10
Weight (kg)						50	50	50	50	50

Superset

	Incline fly					Morey squeeze (upper)				
Sets	1.	2.	3.	4.	5.	1.	2.	3.	4.	5.
Reps	12	10	8	6	4	12	10	8	6	4
Weight (lb)	35	35	35	35	35	20	20	20	20	20

My notes: felt really strong today so I went all out and even managed to bench press 100kg. Felt a really good pump on my lats, chest and even my biceps. With all the weights I give it 100 per cent even if I'm lifting heavy weights and find it difficult.

YOUR TRAINING SESSION

AM

PM Training session Weights – Chest and back

Time trained

Session time

RPE /10

WORKOUT

Deadlift
1 × 20 warm-up – with just Olympic bar

Set and Rep:	1.	2.	3.	4.	5.
Weight (kg):					

Bench press

Set and Rep:	1.	2.	3.	4.	5.
Weight (kg):					

Superset

	Pull-ups (regular)					Low pull				
Sets	1.	2.	3.	4.	5.	1.	2.	3.	4.	5.
Reps										
Weight (kg)										

Superset

	Incline fly					Morey squeeze (upper)				
Sets	1.	2.	3.	4.	5.	1.	2.	3.	4.	5.
Reps										
Weight (kg)										

Your notes:

TRAINING SESSION **WEEK 5** DAY 3

MY TRAINING SESSION

AM Rest

PM Training session CV – Run

Time trained 6.10–6.46 p.m.

Session time 36 minutes

RPE 6/10

WORKOUT
Run – 6 miles
Actual distance: 4.25 miles
Time: 35.58 minutes
Average Pace: 8.28 m/m

My notes: I ran with my dog today, which was the reason I had to stop short on my six-mile run. Unfortunately my dog started to find the pace hard at around three miles, so I headed back home. On the plus side it was one of those runs you think you could carry on forever, so I can't wait for the next run. The terrain was slightly different. I ran in the sea and along some pebbles for around 0.5 miles, which was great fun.

YOUR TRAINING SESSION

AM

PM Training session CV – Run

Time trained

Session time

RPE /10

WORKOUT
Run – 6 miles
Actual distance: miles
Time: minutes
Average Pace: m/m

Your notes:

TRAINING SESSION **WEEK 5** DAY 4

MY TRAINING SESSION

AM Rest

PM Training session CV – Run PT

Time trained 5.40–6.40 p.m.

Session time 1 hour

RPE 4/10

WORKOUT

Run for a mile then get to station 1, complete all the sets and reps for the first exercise, then move on to the next exercise and complete in the same manner. Once you have completed the final exercise at that station, run as fast as you can to the next station to complete those exercises in the same way.

Run 1 mile to station 1
Pull-ups (any): 3 × 15
Sit-ups incline: 3 × 20
½ sit-ups: 3 × 20

Run to station 2
Press-ups: 3 × 30
Pull-ups – regular: 3 × 10

Run to station 3
Dips: 3 × 10
Step-ups: 3 × 20

Run to station 4
Frog hops (as high as possible): 4 × 10

Run 1 mile to finish
Actual distance: 4.32 miles

My notes: I ran with a friend today after work which I hadn't planned to do. I ran approximately 0.75 miles between the fitness stations. The run was slow due to my friend, but that's what made it fun.

YOUR TRAINING SESSION

AM

PM Training session CV – Run PT

Time trained

Session time

RPE /10

WORKOUT

Run 1 mile to station 1
Pull-ups (any): ×
Sit-ups incline: ×
½ sit-ups: ×

Run to station 2
Press-ups: ×
Pull-ups – regular: ×

Run to station 3
Dips: ×
Step-ups: ×

Run to station 4
Frog hops (as high as possible): ×

Run 1 mile to finish
Actual distance: miles

Your notes:

TRAINING SESSION **WEEK 5** DAY 5

MY TRAINING SESSION

AM Training session CV – Walk

Time trained 8.00–10.00 a.m.

Session time 2 hours

RPE 2/10

PM Training session CV – Cycle PT

Time trained 6.10–7.10 p.m.

Session time 1 hour

RPE 8/10

YOUR TRAINING SESSION

AM Training session CV – Walk

Time trained

Session time

RPE /10

PM Training session CV – Cycle PT

Time trained

Session time

RPE /10

WORKOUT
Walk – 2 miles

Cycle PT
There are no reps or sets for the exercises. Perform an exercise while your training partner cycles (sprints) a distance of 400m, and when they get back swap over. When you get back from the cycle, move on to the next exercise. If you're doing this on your own, time your cycle and work all your exercises off that time.

Cycle 1 (repeat twice)
Dumbbell press
Press-ups
300m × cycle sprint
200m × run sprint

Cycle 2 (repeat twice)
Bent-over row
½ sit-ups
Reverse curls

WORKOUT
Walk – 2 miles

Cycle PT

Cycle 2 (repeat twice)
Dumbbell press
Press-ups
300m × cycle sprint
200m × run sprint

Cycle 2 (repeat twice)
Bent-over row
½ sit-ups
Reverse curls

300m × cycle sprint
200m × run sprint

Cycle 3 – legs (repeat three times)
Squats: × 15
Static lunges: × 15
Frog jumps: × 10
Jump overs: × 15
Calf raises: × 15

Cycle 4 – abs
½ sit-ups: × 100
Reverse curls: × 100
Dorsal raise: × 100

My notes: I did this circuit with four friends, which made it really enjoyable. By the end of the day I knew I had worked my legs and glutes.

300m × cycle sprint
200m × run sprint

Cycle 3 – legs (repeat three times)
Squats: ×
Static lunges: ×
Frog jumps: ×
Jump overs: ×
Calf raises: ×

Cycle 4 – abs
½ sit-ups: ×
Reverse curls: ×
Dorsal raise: ×

Your notes:

TRAINING SESSION **WEEK 5** DAY 6

MY TRAINING SESSION

AM Rest

PM Training session Weights – Legs

Time trained 6.15–7.25 p.m.

Session time 1 hour 10 minutes

RPE 8/10

WORKOUT
Squats
1 × 20 warm-up – with just Olympic bar
Set and Rep: 1. 16   2. 16   3. 14   4. 12   5. 12
Weight (lb):   50   70   70   90   90

Stiff leg deadlifts
Set and Rep: 1. 12   2. 12   3. 12
Weight (kg):   55   55   55

Static lunges (dumbbells)
Set and Rep: 1. 12   2. 12   3. 12
Weight (lb):   55   55   55

Calf raises
Set and Rep: 1. 20   2. 20   3. 20   4. 20
Weight (kg):   90   90   90   90

My notes: the squats were really hard half-way through the sets. I had to hydrate quite a lot. My glutes and abs were aching slightly from yesterday's cycle PT, but it's not too bad.

YOUR TRAINING SESSION

AM

PM Training session Weights – Legs

Time trained

Session time

RPE   /10

WORKOUT
Squats
1 × 20 warm-up – with just Olympic bar
Set and Rep: 1.   2.   3.   4.   5.
Weight (kg):

Stiff leg deadlifts
Set and Rep: 1.   2.   3.
Weight (kg):

Static lunges (dumbbells)
Set and Rep: 1.   2.   3.
Weight (kg):

Calf raises
Set and Rep: 1.   2.   3.   4.
Weight (kg):

Your notes:

WEEK 5 TESTS

Front view of me at the end of week 5.

Back view of me at the end of week 5.

MY WEEKLY TESTS

Weight (kg):   80
Height (cm):   175.5
BMI: 26
RHR: 50
BP: 148/53
Fat %:   14.7

Measurements (cm)
Neck: 38.73
Chest: 104.77
Arm: R 36.83   L 36.83
Navel: 82.55
Hips: 86.36
Thighs: R 60.96   L 60.96
Calves: R 40   L 40

YOUR WEEKLY TESTS

Weight (kg):
Height (cm):
BMI:
RHR:
BP:
Fat %:

Measurements (cm)
Neck:
Chest:
Arm: R   L
Navel:
Hips:
Thighs: R   L
Calves: R   L

WEEK SIX NUTRITION PLAN **WEEK 6**

WEEK 6 OVERVIEW

Day	Breakfast	Lunch	Dinner
1	Fruit porridge	Chicken salad	Spicy prawns
2	Wheat biscuits or muesli with fruit	Vegetable soup	Greek chicken salad
3	Muesli with fresh fruit	Chicken wrap	Lamb with rosemary and garlic
4	Fruit smoothie 2	Tuna salad	Butternut squash and spinach frittata
5	Fresh fruit and seeds	Turkey and pine nut salad	Green fish curry
6	Omelette	Rice and salad with beetroot	Beef in black bean sauce
7	Fruit salad	Butternut squash and coriander soup	Kedgeree

SHOPPING LIST **WEEK 6**

CARBOHYDRATES
1 bag of black beans
1 bag of brown basmati rice
1 bag of brown rice
1 bag of wild rice
1 tin of chickpeas
1 bag of long grain rice
250g of muesli
320g porridge oats
1 bag of rice noodles
1 bag of sunflower seeds
1 bag of pumpkin seeds
4 organic tortilla wraps
1 bag of pine nuts
8 Maris piper potatoes
4 sweet potatoes
225g water chestnuts
8 wholemeal/brown pitta
   breads
Wheat biscuits

DAIRY AND NON-DAIRY ALTERNATIVES
200g feta/goat's cheese
50g goat's cheese
17 eggs
1.88 litres skimmed/soya/
   rice/oat milk
2kg soya yoghurt

FISH
225g haddock fillets
225g smoked haddock fillets
700g cooked prawns
4 tinned tuna cans
225g × 4 white fish

MEAT
400g rump beef
8 chicken breasts
400g lean ham
1.5kg leg of lamb
4 turkey breasts

FRUIT
7 apples
2 apricots
6 bananas
1 punnet of blackberries
1 punnet of blueberries
4 lemons
4 peaches
1 large pineapple
1 punnet of raspberries

VEGETABLES

1 avocado
115g baby corn
300g baby spinach
4 cooked beetroot
12 black olives
225g broccoli
1.4kg butternut squash
6 cherry tomatoes
4 carrots
4 celery sticks
1 cos lettuce
1 courgette
2 cucumbers
1 green pepper
2 leeks
2 lettuces
50g mangetout
3 onions
8 plum tomatoes
2 red onions
3 red peppers
8 red tomatoes
175g rocket salad
4 shallots
20 spring onions
1 turnip
3 yellow peppers

HERBS
Basil
Black pepper
Chilli powder
Coriander
Ground coriander
Coriander seeds
Ground
Fresh ginger
2 green chillies
1 garlic bulb
Mint
Nutmeg
Paprika
Parsley
4 red chillies
Rosemary
Turmeric

OTHER
Balsamic vinegar
Brown sugar
150ml coconut milk
Chicken stock
Chinese rice wine
Cold-pressed extra virgin
   olive oil
Peanut oil
Soy sauce
Tahini
800g tinned tomatoes
Vegetable stock
115ml white wine

SNACKS
Fruit
Wholegrain crispbread
   crackers
Flat breads
Small bowl of muesli
Yoghurt/soya yoghurt
Nuts (cashew, pine or
   occasionally mixed nuts)
Soya nuts
Seeds (pumpkin or sunflower)

FRUIT DRINKS
1 carton fruit juice

RECIPES **WEEK 6** DAY 1

BREAKFAST FRUIT PORRIDGE

See page 81

LUNCH CHICKEN SALAD

Cooked chicken from previous night, cut into pieces

Generous amount of salad leaves

1 red pepper, sliced

1 yellow pepper, sliced

2 spring onions, finely chopped

1 Prepare the salad and place chicken over the top.
2 Serve immediately.

DINNER SPICY PRAWNS

2 garlic cloves, finely chopped

2cm piece of fresh ginger, thinly sliced

4 fresh red chillies, deseeded and finely chopped

Olive oil, 1 tablespoon

4 spring onions, chopped

Rice and vegetables of your choice

2 green peppers, deseeded and sliced

400g tin tomatoes

½ tablespoon brown sugar

700g cooked prawns, peeled

4 spring onions, finely sliced to garnish

1 Heat the olive oil in a large wok or frying pan over medium heat.
2 Add ginger, chilli and garlic, stir constantly for 1 minute – do not brown.
3 Add the spring onions and green peppers, stir for 5 minutes.
4 Add the tinned tomatoes and sugar, bring to boil and stir constantly. If sauce is too thick, add a little water.
5 Reduce heat and simmer for 5 minutes.
6 Stir in the prawns and cook for 4 minutes.
7 Transfer food to plates, garnish with spring onions and serve with rice/vegetables.

Lunch for tomorrow:
VEGETABLE SOUP
See the following page and consider preparing your lunch in advance.

RECITS **WEEK 6** DAY 2

BREAKFAST WHEAT BISCUITS
OR MUESLI WITH FRUIT

See page 84

LUNCH VEGETABLE SOUP

See page 100

DINNER GREEK CHICKEN SALAD

1 cos lettuce, cut into large pieces

1 cucumber, roughly chopped

1 green pepper, deseeded and finely chopped

12 olives (optional)

½ red onion, finely sliced

8 plum tomatoes

1 tablespoon lemon juice

1 tablespoon olive oil

200g low fat feta/goat's cheese

4 chicken breasts

8 wholemeal pitta breads (2 per person)

For the tzatziki:

1 clove of garlic, crushed

200g soya/plain yoghurt

¼ cucumber, finely grated

½ small red onion, finely chopped

1 tablespoon parsley, chopped

1 tablespoon mint, chopped

For the humous:

1 large tin chickpeas, drained

2 cloves garlic, peeled

2–3 tablespoons olive oil

1 dessertspoon tahini

1 Put the lettuce, cucumber, pepper, olives, tomatoes and onion into a large salad bowl.
2 Add the olive oil and lemon juice and mix well.
3 Crumble the feta/goat's cheese or mature goat's cheese over the top.
4 Prepare the tzatziki by mixing all the ingredients together in a small bowl.
5 Prepare humous by placing all the ingredients in a blender and blend until a smooth paste.
6 Meanwhile, grill the chicken on a medium heat for 8–12 minutes, or until thoroughly cooked.
7 Allow to cool for a couple of minutes and cut into pieces.
8 Toast the pitta bread before serving then fill with chicken, salad, tzatziki and humous.

Lunch for tomorrow:
CHICKEN WRAP
Consider preparing extra chicken in advance for tomorrow's lunch (refrigerate overnight).

RECIPES **WEEK 6** DAY 3

BREAKFAST MUESLI WITH FRESH FRUIT

See page 80

LUNCH CHICKEN WRAP

See page 113

DINNER LAMB WITH ROSEMARY AND GARLIC

1.5kg lean leg of lamb (200g per person)
1 tablespoon olive oil
2 sprigs rosemary
2 cloves garlic, peeled and halved
2 lemons, quartered
115ml white wine

Serve with your favourite vegetables or beans and 8 roast potatoes (2 per person)

1 Preheat oven to 180°C (350°F).
2 Rub meat with olive oil.
3 Place rosemary, garlic and lemon in a baking dish and pour in the white wine.
4 Add lamb on top and bake for 1 to 1½ hours depending on taste.
5 Cook your vegetables and roast the potatoes.
6 Remove from oven, cover with foil and set aside for 10 minutes before carving.

**Lunch for tomorrow:
TUNA SALAD**
Consider preparing sweet potatoes in advance for tomorrow's lunch.

RECITPES **WEEK 6** DAY 4

BREAKFAST FRUIT SMOOTHIE 2   *See page 152*

LUNCH TUNA SALAD   *See page 131*

DINNER BUTTERNUT SQUASH AND SPINACH FRITTATA

400g butternut squash, peeled and cut into 3cm cubes

1 tablespoon olive oil

1 teaspoon soy sauce

2 leeks, finely chopped and washed

2 cloves garlic, crushed

300g baby spinach

8 eggs

400g soya/plain yoghurt

50g matured/goat's cheese, grated

Salad leaves

1 Preheat oven to 170°C (330°F). Grease a small baking dish with a little olive oil.
2 Place butternut squash in baking tray, add 1 teaspoon of olive oil and soy sauce and roast for 25 minutes.
3 Heat the rest of the olive oil over a medium heat.
4 Add the leek and cook for 5 minutes, or until soft. Then add the garlic and spinach leaves and cook until spinach has wilted.
5 Whisk eggs, soya/plain yoghurt and cheese together in large bowl.
6 Then add the butternut squash and spinach mixture and gently stir.
7 Pour the mixture into a baking dish and cook for 20 minutes, or until set. Serve with salad.

Lunch for tomorrow:
TURKEY AND PINE NUT SALAD
Consider preparing turkey breasts in advance for tomorrow's lunch.

RECIPES **WEEK 6** DAY 5

BREAKFAST FRESH FRUIT AND SEEDS

See page 82

LUNCH TURKEY AND PINE NUT SALAD

½ tablespoon olice oil

3–4 tablespoons of pine nuts

4 cooked turkey breasts, cut into pieces

Generous amount of salad leaves

1 avocado, sliced

1 red pepper, sliced

1 yellow pepper, sliced

2 spring onions, finely chopped

1 Heat the olive oil in a frying pan over a medium heat.
2 Cook the turkey breasts for 8–10 minutes, or until cooked.
3 Allow turkey to cool.
4 Prepare the salad and arrange the cooked turkey on top of the leaves.
5 Sprinkle with the pine nuts.
6 Drizzle with balsamic vinegar and serve immediately.

DINNER GREEN FISH CURRY

1 tablespoon olive oil

2 spring onions, sliced

1 teaspoon ground cumin seeds

2 green chillies, finely chopped

1 teaspoon coriander seeds

4 tablespoons fresh coriander

4 tablespoons fresh mint

150ml coconut milk

4 white fish fillets (225g each)

Rice and/or vegetables

1 Heat the olive oil in a large frying pan over a medium heat. Add the spring onions and cook for 2 minutes or until soft.
2 Stir in ground cumin, chillies and coriander seeds and cook until the spices are fragrant.
3 Add the fresh coriander, mint, and coconut milk.
4 Carefully cook fish in frying pan 10–15 minutes or until the flesh flakes easily when tested with a fork.
5 Transfer the fish on to plates and serve with rice and vegetables of your choice.
6 Garnish with fresh mint.

**Dinner for tomorrow:
BEEF IN BLACK BEAN SAUCE**
Consider preparing marinade in advance (leave in fridge to marinate overnight).

RECIPES **WEEK 6** DAY 6

BREAKFAST OMELETTE

See page 88

LUNCH RICE AND SALAD WITH BEETROOT

100g brown rice

100g wild rice

4 shallots, peeled and halved

2 teaspoons olive oil

4 cooked beetroots, finely diced

1 lemon, juice of

2 tablespoons fresh mint, chopped

2 tablespoons fresh parsley, chopped

1 Preheat oven to 200°C (400°F). Place brown and wild rice in saucepan of water, bring to boil and simmer for 20 minutes.
2 Place the shallots on a baking tray, drizzle with olive oil and roast for 8–10 minutes.
3 Drain the rice and allow to cool. Mix the beetroot, lemon juice and mint. Stir in shallots and parsley, then serve.

DINNER BEEF IN BLACK BEAN SAUCE

400g lean rump steak, remove fat, cut into chunks

1 tablespoon olive oil

225g broccoli, cut into florets

115g baby corns, cut in half

4 spring onions, sliced diagonally

225g tinned water chestnuts

Rice or egg noodles

For the marinade:

1 tablespoon black beans, soaked in cold water for 5–10 minutes

2 tablespoons dark soy sauce

2 tablespoons Chinese rice wine

1 tablespoon peanut oil

1 teaspoon brown sugar

1 garlic clove, thinly sliced

1 tablespoon ginger, finely chopped

1 To make marinade: mash black beans in a bowl with a fork, stir in the remaining marinade ingredients and blend with a food processor.
2 Pour the marinade over steak and coat thoroughly in a baking dish. Cover with cling film and leave in fridge for 6 hours or more.
3 Heat the olive oil in large wok or frying pan. Drain the steak and reserve the marinade.
4 Stir fry the steak over a medium/high heat for 3 minutes, then transfer to a plate.
5 Add the broccoli and baby corn to the wok and stir in 3 tablespoons of water, cover and steam for 5 minutes, or until the vegetables are tender.
6 Add spring onions and water chestnuts to the wok and stir fry for a further 2 minutes.
7 Return the steak to the wok and pour in the reserved marinade.
8 Cook and keep stirring, until heated through. Serve with noodles of your choice.

RECIPES **WEEK 6** DAY 7

BREAKFAST FRUIT SALAD   *See page 85*

LUNCH BUTTERNUT SQUASH AND CORIANDER SOUP   *See page 88*

DINNER KEDGEREE

225g haddock fillet
225g smoked haddock fillet
1 tablespoon olive oil
1 onion, chopped
225g long grain rice
1 hard-boiled egg, cut into quarters
2 tablespoons fresh parsley
Spices:
½ teaspoon ground turmeric
½ teaspoon cumin
½ teaspoon chilli powder
¼ teaspoon ground ginger

1 Place the haddock and smoked haddock in large frying pan.
2 Pour enough water to cover, and poach gently over a low heat for 10–15 minutes.
3 Remove from heat and allow to cool.
4 Sieve the cooking liquid into a measuring jug and make it up to 600ml if necessary.
5 Heat the olive oil in a large frying pan.
6 Add the onions and cook on low heat for 3 minutes, or until soft.
7 Mix in the spices, add the rice and cook. Stir until well coated.
8 Gently stir in the reserved liquid and bring to boil.
9 Cover and cook over low heat for 20 minutes, or until the liquid has been absorbed into the rice.
10 Meanwhile, skin the fish and remove any remaining bones.
11 Flake the flesh and fold the fish into the rice.
12 Transfer to a serving dish and garnish with a boiled egg.
13 Sprinkle over the chopped parsley and serve immediately.

TRAINING DIARY **WEEK 6**

WEEK 6 OVERVIEW
Day 1: Weights – Chest and back
Day 2: CV – Run PT
Day 3: CV – Run; Weights – Shoulders and arms
Day 4: Weights – Legs
Day 5: PT – Upper body
Day 6: Circuits
Day 7: Rest
Any day: Myo stretch

MY DIARY
Day 1 (Monday)
I had a nice long lie in with Alison. She then took me on one of my favourite special walks. We ended up walking for over four hours and had lunch out.
Tiredness 1
Stress 1
Sleep 7 hours

Day 2 (Tuesday)
Worked at Poole today and when I finished I went for a run around Poole Park where they have new circuit equipment.
Tiredness 5
Stress 4
Sleep 6 hours

Day 3 (Wednesday)
Trained after work. Chilled out tonight with some friends who came over.
Tiredness 4
Stress 4
Sleep 7 hours

Day 4 (Thursday)
I'm aching a little bit today after training yesterday. I ended up getting talked into going out with my friends till 12.30 a.m. I only had one drink, and by the time I got into bed I was feeling shattered.
Tiredness 6
Stress 4
Sleep 6 hours

Day 5 (Friday)
Still aching and feeling slightly tender in some of my muscles, but in a good way. I had another late night but it was my own fault as I got stuck into changing the interior of my house around.
Tiredness 4
Stress 3
Sleep 7 hours

Day 6 (Saturday)
Spent the day with Alison. We went for a nice romantic walk along the beach.
Tiredness 3
Stress 3
Sleep 4 hours 30 minutes

Day 7 (Sunday)
Day off. Went and had a synaesthesia massage again.
Tiredness 3
Stress 3
Sleep 4 hours 30 minutes

TRAINING SESSION **WEEK 6** DAY 1

MY TRAINING SESSION

AM Rest

PM **Training session** Weights – Chest and back

Time trained 5.40–7.15 p.m.

Session time 1 hour 35 minutes

RPE 6/10

WORKOUT
Exercise cycle
Perform all of the exercises below with 30 reps in number order.
1. Step-up
2. Dumbbell press
3. Crunches
4. Box jumps
5. Bent-over row
6. Reverse curl

Bench press
1 × 20 warm-up – with just Olympic bar

Set and Rep:	1. 10	2. 10	3. 10	4. 7	5. 8	6. 6
Weight (kg):	40	60	90	100	100	105

Superset

	Bent-over row			Incline flyers		
Sets and Reps	1. 10	2. 10	3. 10	1. 10	2. 10	3. 10
Weight (kg)	75	75	75	55	55	55

Morey squeeze (upper)

Set and Rep:	1. 10	2. 10	3. 10
Weight (lb):	22.5	22.5	22.5

YOUR TRAINING SESSION

AM

PM **Training session** Weights – Chest and back

Time trained

Session time

RPE /10

WORKOUT
Exercise cycle

1. Step-up
2. Dumbbell press
3. Crunches
4. Box jumps
5. Bent-over row
6. Reverse curl

Bench press
1 × 20 warm-up – with just Olympic bar

Set and Rep:	1.	2.	3.	4.	5.	6.
Weight (kg):						

Superset

	Bent-over row			Incline flyers		
Set and Rep:	1.	2.	3.	1.	2.	3.
Weight (kg):						

Morey squeeze (upper)

Set and Rep:	1.	2.	3.
Weight (kg):			

Reverse shrug

Set and Rep:	1. 10	2. 10	3. 10	4. 10
Weight (kg):	75	75	75	75

Bent-over lat raise

Set and Rep:	1. 10	2. 10	3. 10	4. 10
Weight (lb):	25	25	25	25

Superset

	Cable cross-over (single side)			*Single arm cable row*		
Sets and Reps	1. 10	2. 10	3. 10	1. 10	2. 10	3. 10
Weight (kg)	10	10	10	20	20	20

My notes: I trained outside in the lovely sunshine. This is quite a slow but intense workout, which makes you believe you could lift more and go on for longer.

Reverse shrug

Set and Rep:	1.	2.	3.	4.
Weight (kg):				

Bent-over lat raise

Set and Rep:	1.	2.	3.	4.
Weight (kg):				

Superset

	Cable cross-over (single side)			*Single arm cable row*		
Set and Rep:	1.	2.	3.	1.	2.	3.
Weight (kg):						

Your notes:

TRAINING SESSION **WEEK 6** DAY 2

MY TRAINING SESSION

AM Rest

PM Training session CV – Run PT

Time trained 5.30–6.30 p.m.

Session time 1 hour

RPE 7/10

YOUR TRAINING SESSION

AM

PM Training session CV – Run PT

Time trained

Session time

RPE /10

WORKOUT

Run for a mile to station 1, then complete all the sets and reps for the first exercise, then move on to the next exercise and complete in the same manner. Once you have completed the final exercise at that station, run as fast as you can to the next station to complete those exercises in the same way.

Run PT
Total distance: 4.32 miles

Run 1 mile to station 1
Pull-ups (any): 3 × 10
Leg levers: 3 × 10
Sit-ups incline: 3 × 20
½ sit-ups: 3 × 20

Run to station 2
Press-ups: 3 × 30
Pull-ups – regular: 3 × 10
Leg levers: 3 × 10

Run to station 3
Dips: 3 × 10
Step-ups: 3 × 20
Press-ups wide: 3 × 20
Press-ups (feet up): 3 × 10

Run to station 4
Frog hops (as high as possible): 4 × 12

Run 1 mile to finish

My notes: I ran approximately 0.75 miles between the fitness stations. Really enjoyed today's training in the sunshine. Ran with the same friend from last time. This time we were both a lot quicker. Finally my muscles don't ache so I was full of beans.

WORKOUT

Run PT
Total distance:

Run 1 mile to station 1
Pull-ups (any):   ×
Leg levers: ×
Sit-ups incline: ×
½ sit-ups: ×

Run to station 2
Press-ups: ×
Pull-ups – regular: ×
Leg levers: ×

Run to station 3
Dips: ×
Step-ups: ×
Press-ups wide: ×
Press-ups (feet up):   ×

Run to station 4
Frog hops (as high as possible):   ×

Run 1 mile to finish

Your notes:

TRAINING SESSION **WEEK 6** DAY 3

MY TRAINING SESSION

AM Rest

PM Training session CV – Run

Time trained 6.52– 7.15 p.m.

Session time 23 minutes

RPE 8/10

PM Training session Weights – Shoulders and arms

Time trained 7.15–8.20 p.m.

Session time 1 hour 5 minutes

RPE 8/10

WORKOUT
Once you have finished the three-mile run go straight into weight training without taking a rest.

Run – 3 miles
Actual distance: 3.05 miles
Time: 22.30 minutes
Average Pace: 7.30 m/m

Military press
1 × 20 warm-up – with just Olympic bar
Set and Rep: 1. 10   2. 10   3. 9   4. 7   5. 6
Weight (kg):   40   50   55   55   55

Arnold press
Set and Rep: 1. 10   2. 8   3. 6   4. 4
Weight (lb):   35   35   35   35

YOUR TRAINING SESSION

AM

PM   Training session CV – Run

Time trained

Session time

RPE   /10

PM   Training session Weights – Shoulders and arms

Time trained

Session time

RPE   /10

WORKOUT

Run – 3 miles
Actual distance: miles
Time: minutes
Average Pace: m/m

Military press
1 × 20 warm-up – with just Olympic bar
Set and Rep: 1.   2.   3.   4.   5.
Weight (kg):

Arnold press
Set and Rep: 1.   2.   3.   4.
Weight (lb):

Bent-over lat raise

Set and Rep:	1. 10	2. 10	3. 10	4. 10
Weight (lb):	17.5	22.5	30	30

Arm curl (Olympic bar)

Set and Rep:	1. 10	2. 10	3. 10	4. 10
Weight (kg):	35	35	35	35

Skull crusher

Set and Rep:	1. 10	2. 10	3. 10	4. 10
Weight (kg):	35	35	35	35

Superset

	Supernated curl				Triceps kickback			
Sets	1.	2.	3.	4.	1.	2.	3.	4
Reps	10	10	10	10	10	10	10	10
Weight (lb)	35	52.5	52.5	52.5	20	30	30	30

My notes: excellent workout. Went for a three-mile run and at the end, at around 0.3 miles before the end, I sprinted. I then went straight into the gym. Felt really strong with the weights and loved the supersets at the end on my arms.

Bent-over lat raise

Set and Rep:	1.	2.	3.	4.
Weight (lb):				

Arm curl (Olympic bar)

Set and Rep:	1.	2.	3.	4.
Weight (kg):				

Skull crusher

Set and Rep:	1.	2.	3.	4.
Weight (kg):				

Superset

	Supernated curl				Triceps kickback			
Sets	1.	2.	3.	4.	1.	2.	3.	4.
Reps								
Weight (kg)								

Your notes:

TRAINING SESSION **WEEK 6** DAY 4

MY TRAINING SESSION

AM Rest

PM Training session Weights – Legs

Time trained 6.00–7.05 p.m.

Session time 1 hour 5 minutes

RPE 7/10

WORKOUT
Squats
1 × 20 warm-up – with just Olympic bar.
Set and Rep: 1. 16   2. 16   3. 16   4. 12   5. 13
Weight (lb):   50   70   90   90   90

Stiff leg deadlifts
Set and Rep: 1. 12   2. 12   3. 12
Weight (kg):   65   65   65

Calf raises
Set and Rep: 1. 20   2. 20   3. 20   4. 20
Weight (kg):   110   110   110   110

Cycle (repeat 3 times)
Lunge jumps (weight 8kg): × 10
Squat jumps (weight 8kg): × 10
Squats bosu (upside down, weight 8kg): × 30

My notes: out of all of the exercises, I find the squats the hardest and again I felt completely knackered. I could have gone heavier with the calf raises, but if I did I would need to buy wrist straps to help me hold the weight.

YOUR TRAINING SESSION

AM

PM Training session Weights – Legs

Time trained

Session time

RPE   /10

WORKOUT
Squats
1 × 20 warm-up – with just Olympic bar
Set and Rep: 1.   2.   3.   4.   5.
Weight (lb):

Stiff leg deadlifts
Set and Rep: 1.   2.   3.
Weight (kg):

Calf raises
Set and Rep: 1.   2.   3.   4.
Weight (kg):

Cycle (repeat 3 times)
Lunge jumps (weight   kg): ×
Squat jumps (weight   kg): ×
Squats bosu (upside down, weight   kg): ×

Your notes:

TRAINING SESSION **WEEK 6** DAY 5

MY TRAINING SESSION

AM Rest

PM **Training session** PT – Upper body

Time trained 5.55–6.40 p.m.

Session time 45 minutes

RPE 7/10

WORKOUT
Complete all the pull-ups first then move on to the chest and abs. Don't rest in between sets and reps on any exercise.

Regular pull-ups
1 – 10 – 10 – 1
Total: 110

Chest and abs cycle (repeat 15 times)
Regular press-ups: × 10
½ sit-ups: × 10
Diamond press-ups: × 10
Leg levers: × 10
Wide push-ups: × 10
V sit-ups: × 10
Total press-ups: 450
Total sit-ups: 450

My notes: the pull-ups were nice and easy but the press-ups and sit-ups were hard. My triceps were still aching from Wednesday. You should enjoy this quick workout.

YOUR TRAINING SESSION

AM

PM **Training session** PT – Upper body

Time trained

Session time

RPE /10

WORKOUT

Regular pull-ups
–   –   –

Total:

Chest and abs cycle (repeat 15 times)
Regular press-ups: ×
½ sit-ups: ×
Diamond press-ups: ×
Leg levers: ×
Wide push-ups: ×
V sit-ups: ×
Total press-ups:
Total sit-ups:

Your notes:

TRAINING SESSION **WEEK 6** DAY 6

MY TRAINING SESSION

AM Rest

PM **Training session** Circuits

Time trained 12.30–1.30 p.m.

Session time 1 hour

RPE 9/10

YOUR TRAINING SESSION

AM

PM **Training session** Circuits

Time trained

Session time

RPE /10

WORKOUT

Below are three different cycles. On cycle 1 and 2, each exercise is timed and lasts for one minute. Complete all the exercises labelled cycle 1 in order, then move on to cycles 2 and 3. All weight exercises use 13kg.

Key AC=Arm curl, BOR=Bent-over row, PF=Pec fly, PO=Pull-overs, SC=Skull crusher, SP=Dumbbell press

Cycle 1

1. Step-up	1. Toe taps	1. Side lunge
2. BOR	2. BOR/SP	2. BOR/SP/AC
3. Step-up	3. Toe taps	3. Side lunge
4. BOR	4. BOR/SP	4. BOR/SP/AC
5. Step-up	5. Toe taps	5. Side lunge
6. BOR	6. BOR/SP	6. BOR/SP/AC

Cycle 2

1. ½ sit-up	1. Leg levers	1. Heel taps
2. PF	2. PF/SC	2. PF/SC/PO
3. ½ sit-up	3. Leg levers	3. Heel taps
4. PF	4. PF/SC	4. PF/SC/PO
5. ½ sit-up	5. Leg levers	5. Heel taps
6. PF	6. PF/SC	6. PF/SC/PO

Cycle 3

1. Skipping: 3 × 1 minute
2. Supernation curl (weight 23kg): 3 × 10
3. Incline Fly (weight 11kg): 3 × 10

My notes: my legs were aching too much to do any type of running or exercises. Go as fast as you can for each minute and you will get an amazing feeling at the end.

WORKOUT

Your notes:

WEEK 6 TESTS

Front view of me at the end of
week 6.

Back view of me at the end of
week 6.

MY WEEKLY TESTS

Weight (kg): 79
Height (cm): 175.5
BMI: 25.6
RHR: 50
BP: 148/48
Fat %: 13.9

Measurements (cm)
Neck: 38.73
Chest: 106.04
Arm: R 36.83   L 36.83
Navel: 80.64
Hips: 83.82
Thighs: R 60.96   L 60.96
Calves: R 40   L 40

YOUR WEEKLY TESTS

Weight (kg):
Height (cm):
BMI:
RHR:
BP:
Fat %:

Measurements (cm)
Neck:
Chest:
Arm: R   L
Navel:
Hips:
Thighs: R   L
Calves: R   L

You are over half-way, so keep on going.

WEEK **SEVEN** NUTRITION PLAN **WEEK 7**

WEEK 7 OVERVIEW

Day	Breakfast	Lunch	Dinner
1	Wheat biscuits or muesli with fruit	Beef salad pitta	Snapper with basil
2	Fruit salad	Yellow split pea soup	Chicken with roasted tomatoes
3	Muesli with fresh fruit	Chicken wrap	Lamb with baked fennel
4	Fruit porridge	Egg salad	Citrus baked cod
5	Fresh fruit and seeds	Tuna salad	Soya/plain yoghurt baked chicken
6	Omelette	Tomato and pepper soup	Vegetarian stir fry
7	Fruit smoothie 1	Salmon salad	Spiced barramundi fillets

SHOPPING LIST **WEEK 7**

CARBOHYDRATES
1 bag of brown rice
12 charlotte potatoes
240g of muesli
560g porridge oats
1 bag of rice noodles
1 bag of sunflower seeds
1 bag of pumpkin seeds
4 organic tortilla wraps
1 bag of sesame seeds
5 sweet potatoes
4 wholemeal/brown pitta
   breads
225g yellow split peas
Wheat biscuits

DAIRY AND NON-DAIRY ALTERNATIVES
12 eggs
60g feta/goat's cheese
680ml skimmed/soya/rice/
   oat milk
2kg soya yoghurt

FISH
200g × 4 barramundi
175g × 4 cod/hake
200g × 4 snapper fillets
4 poached salmon fillets
4 small tins tuna

MEAT
400g cooked roast beef
12 chicken breasts
400g lean ham
1.4kg lamb cutlets

FRUIT
3 apples
4 bananas
2 lemons
2 limes
2 mangos
1 melon
1 orange
1 large pineapple
1 punnet of raspberries

VEGETABLES
100g baby corn
3 bags of baby spinach
55g button mushrooms
1 broccoli floret
350g cabbage
400g cherry tomatoes
3 carrots
1 courgette
2 cucumbers
2 fennel bulbs
1 green pepper
4 lettuce
200g mangetout
150g mushrooms
6 onions
2 red onions
4 red peppers
100g rocket salad
20g snow pea pods
11 spring onions
750g tomatoes
21 red tomatoes
5 yellow peppers

HERBS
Basil
Black pepper
Cardamom seeds
Chilli powder
Chinese five-spice
Cinnamon
Coriander
Cumin
Fresh ginger
1 garlic bulb
Mint
Oregano
Parsley
1 red chilli
Rosemary
Tarragon

OTHER
Balsamic vinegar
Cider vinegar
Cold-pressed extra virgin
   olive oil
Dijon mustard
Oyster sauce
Peanut oil
Sesame oil
Soy sauce
Tomato purée
Vegetable stock
60ml white wine

SNACKS
Wholegrain crispbread
   crackers
Crackers/flat breads
Small bowl of muesli
Yoghurt/soya yoghurt
Nuts (cashew, pine or
   occasionally mixed nuts)
Soya nuts
Seeds (pumpkin or sunflower)

FRUIT DRINKS
1 carton fruit juice

RECIPES **WEEK 7** DAY 1

BREAKFAST WHEAT BISCUITS OR MUESLI WITH FRUIT

See page 84

LUNCH BEEF SALAD PITTA

See page 101

DINNER SNAPPER WITH BASIL

4 × 200g snapper fillets
2 tablespoons olive oil
1 clove garlic, crushed
½ red chilli, finely chopped
4 spring onions, finely chopped
2 tablespoons basil, roughly chopped
1 tablespoon dried oregano
60ml white wine
4 tomatoes, roughly chopped
Green salas

1. Preheat oven to 180°C (350°F).
2. Heat half the olive oil in a small saucepan over a medium heat.
3. Add the chilli, garlic and spring onions and stir fry for 2 minutes, or until garlic is golden.
4. Reduce the heat to medium low and add the herbs and white wine, stirring occasionally for 5 minutes.
5. Remove from heat and stir in the chopped tomatoes.
6. Heat a large non-stick frying pan over a high heat and brush the fish with the remaining oil.
7. Sear each side for 2 minutes and transfer to an ovenproof baking dish and spoon sauce over fish.
8. Bake for 6–8 minutes or until fish is cooked. The flesh will flake away easily when pressed with a fork when the fish is ready. Serve with salad.

Lunch for tomorrow:
YELLOW SPLIT PEA SOUP
Soak the yellow split peas overnight for tomorrow's lunch.

RECIPES **WEEK 7** DAY 2

BREAKFAST FRUIT SALAD   *See page 85*

LUNCH YELLOW SPLIT PEA SOUP   *See page 146*

DINNER CHICKEN WITH ROASTED TOMATOES

4 large tomatoes, cut into quarters

1 tablespoon olive oil

1 small onion, sliced

1 tablespoon fresh basil, roughly chopped

4 × 200g skinless chicken breasts

60g goat's or mature cheese, cut into chunks

Salad or vegetables of your choice

1 Preheat oven to 180°C (350°F). Line a baking tray with baking paper and place tomatoes on tray.
2 Place in a hot oven for 15 minutes. Meanwhile, heat the olive oil in a frying pan over medium heat.
3 Add the onion and basil and cook for 5 minutes or until onion is soft.
4 Drain and reserve the oil and place onion and basil on a plate.
5 Return pan to heat and add the reserved oil.
6 Add chicken and cook for 6 minutes each side, or until lightly browned on both sides.
7 Heat grill to medium.
8 Divide the chicken into four portions and cover the chicken with a layer of the tomato and onion mixture.
9 Top with feta/goat's cheese and place under grill until the cheese has melted.
10 Serve with either salad or vegetables.

Lunch for tomorrow:
CHICKEN WRAP
Consider preparing extra chicken in advance for tomorrow's lunch.

RECITES **WEEK 7** DAY 3

BREAKFAST MUESLI WITH
FRESH FRUIT

See page 80

LUNCH CHICKEN WRAP

See page 113

DINNER LAMB WITH
BAKED FENNEL

1.4kg lamb cutlets (200g meat per person)
with fat trimmed off

2 fennel bulbs, sliced

2 red onions, cut into wedges

1 tablespoon olive oil

100g baby spinach leaves

8–12 Charlotte potatoes

For the marinade:

2 tablespoons rosemary, chopped

2 teaspoons tarragon, chopped

2 teaspoons parsley

1 tablespoon olive oil

1 Mix the marinade ingredients together and pour into a shallow dish.
2 Add the meat to the marinade and coat thoroughly.
3 Cover and allow to marinate for 30 minutes.
4 Preheat oven to 180°C (350°F).
5 Place fennel and onion in a baking dish and drizzle with olive oil and bake for 20 minutes.
6 Roast the potatoes.
7 Preheat grill to high and cook the lamb cutlets to your liking.
8 Once cooked, set aside to rest. Toss the spinach leaves through the hot vegetables.
9 Arrange the vegetables on serving plates and place the lamb on top.
10 Serve with potatoes.

Lunch for tomorrow:
EGG SALAD
Consider preparing eggs in advance (refrigerate overnight).

RECIPES **WEEK 7** DAY 4

BREAKFAST FRUIT PORRIDGE   *See page 81*

LUNCH EGG SALAD   *See page 116*

DINNER CITRUS BAKED COD

4 × cod or hake cutlets (175g/6oz each)

2 tablespoons lime juice

1 green pepper, deseeded and cut into strips

1 tablespoon olive oil

1 onion, finely chopped

1 clove garlic, crushed

40g pumpkin seeds

1 lime, grated zest

1 tablespoon coriander, chopped

55g button mushrooms, finely sliced

2 tablespoons fresh orange juice or white wine

Broccoli

1 Place fish in a shallow ovenproof dish and pour over lime juice.
2 Cover and leave to marinade in the refrigerator for 15–25 minutes.
3 Preheat oven to 180°C (350°F).
4 Heat olive oil in a frying pan and cook onion, garlic, green pepper and pumpkin seeds. Cook until onion is soft.
5 Gently stir in the lime zest, chopped coriander and mushrooms.
6 Spoon this mixture over fish and pour over the orange juice.
7 Cover and bake in oven for 30 minutes, or until fish is tender.
8 Serve with steamed broccoli.

**Lunch for tomorrow:
TUNA SALAD**
Consider preparing sweet potatoes for tomorrow's lunch in advance.

RECIPES **WEEK 7** DAY 5

BREAKFAST FRESH FRUIT AND SEEDS

See page 82

LUNCH TUNA SALAD

See page 131

DINNER SOYA/PLAIN YOGHURT BAKED CHICKEN

1 tablespoon olive oil

4 × 200g skinless chicken breasts

For the salad:

½ cucumber, sliced

4 large tomatoes, sliced

½ small red onion, finely sliced

½ tablespoon mint leaves

1 teaspoon lemon juice

For the marinade:

½ teaspoon Chinese five-spice powder

1 teaspoon chilli powder

2 teaspoons soy sauce

1 glove garlic, crushed

1 tablespoon olive oil

200g soya/plain yoghurt

1 In a bowl fold the five-spice powder, chilli powder, soy sauce, garlic and olive oil through the soya/plain yoghurt.
2 Coat the chicken with the mixture and leave to marinate for up to 4 hours.
3 Preheat the oven to 180°C (350°F).
4 Line a baking dish with baking paper.
5 Heat the olive oil in a non-stick frying pan over medium heat.
6 Add the chicken and cook for 2 minutes each side.
7 Transfer the chicken to the prepared baking dish and bake for 6–8 minutes or until cooked.
8 Remove from oven and allow to rest for 5 minutes.
9 Cut into thick slices.
10 Prepare the salad adding all the ingredients in salad bowl and mix.
11 Serve salad with the chicken.

RECIPES **WEEK 7** DAY 6

BREAKFAST OMELETTE   *See page 88*

LUNCH TOMATO AND PEPPER SOUP   *See page 135*

DINNER VEGETARIAN STIR FRY

1 tablespoon peanut oil

1 clove garlic

1 teaspoon ginger, grated

1 onion, sliced

150g mangetout

150g mushrooms

350g cabbage, shredded

100g baby corn

2 tablespoons oyster sauce

1 tablespoon soy sauce

2 tablespoons coriander leaves

Brown rice

1   Heat a large wok or frying pan over high heat.
2   Add peanut oil, and once pan is smoking add the garlic, ginger and onion.
3   Stir fry for 2–3 minutes or until the onion begins to soften.
4   Next, add the mangetout, mushrooms, cabbage and baby corn and stir fry for a further 5 minutes, or until almost cooked.
5   Add the oyster sauce, soy sauce and coriander and cook for 1 minute.
6   Serve immediately with brown rice.

RECIPES **WEEK 7** DAY 7

BREAKFAST FRUIT SMOOTHIE 1   *See page 87*

LUNCH SALMON SALAD   *See page 118*

DINNER SPICED BARRAMUNDI STEAKS

1 tablespoon olive oil

4 × 200g barramundi fillets

1 tablespoon sesame oil

20g snow pea pods (string removed)

1 tablespoon sesame seeds

1 large yellow pepper, cut into thin strips

Brown rice

For the paste:

Freshly ground pepper

1 teaspoon ground cumin

½ teaspoon ground cardamom

½ teaspoon ground cinnamon

1 clove garlic, chopped

1 tablespoon fresh coriander

1 tablespoon parsley

1 lemon, juice and finely grated zest

1 Preheat oven to 180°C (350°F). Pat fish with paper towel, brush with half the olive oil and season.
2 Place fish in a single layer in an ovenproof baking dish.
3 Next, mix the remaining olive oil with the cumin, coriander, cardamom, cinnamon, garlic, parsley, and lemon juice and zest until you have a loose paste and spread evenly over the top of the fish.
4 Cover dish with foil and bake for 10–15 minutes, or until fish is cooked. Boil the rice.
5 Heat the sesame oil over medium to high heat and add the snow pea pods and sesame seeds.
6 Cook for 2 minutes or until snow pea pods are crisp tender. Gently stir in the yellow pepper and cook for a further 2 minutes. Serve immediately with barramundi and rice.

Lunch for tomorrow:
SWEET POTATO AND BEAN SALAD
Consider preparing eggs and sweet potatoes in advance (refrigerate overnight).

TRAINING DIARY **WEEK 7**

WEEK 7 OVERVIEW
Day 1: CV – Run
Day 2: Weights – Chest and back
Day 3: CV – Run
Day 4: Weights – Shoulders and arms
Day 5: PT – Lower body
Day 6: Circuits
Day 7: Rest
Any day: Myo stretch

MY DIARY
Day 1 (Monday)
I went for a really nice run in the rain – no surprise that I saw no one else out and about.
Tiredness 4
Stress 3
Sleep 6 hours 45 minutes

Day 2 (Tuesday)
Nothing interesting happened today.
Tiredness 4
Stress 4
Sleep 6 hours

Day 3 (Wednesday)
I am feeling really good at the moment and I am definitely seeing a lot of results.
Tiredness 3
Stress 3
Sleep 6 hours

Day 4 (Thursday)
Trained late today, as I was undecided about whether or not I should train, my mind was saying yes but the body was saying no. I did eventually get out there – you have to push yourself from time to time.
Tiredness 5
Stress 3
Sleep 7 hours

Day 5 (Friday)
I had a little bit of work in the morning before spending the evening with Alison.
Tiredness 3
Stress 2
Sleep 6 hours 30 minutes

Day 6 (Saturday)
Went for a two-mile walk, and the rest of my spare time was attempting to do the garden, which I felt was quite hard work.
Tiredness 2
Stress 2
Sleep 7 hours 30 minutes

Day 7 (Sunday)
My older brother came down from London to stay the night. It was nice as he noticed the change in my physique. He even commented about my lack of spots.
Tiredness 3
Stress 2
Sleep 7 hours

TRAINING SESSION **WEEK 7** DAY 1

MY TRAINING SESSION

AM Rest

PM **Training session** CV – Run

Time trained 6.05–7.00 p.m.

Session time 55 minutes

RPE 5/10

WORKOUT
Run – 6 miles
Actual distance: 6.02 miles
Time: 51.53 minutes
Average pace: 8.37 m/m

My notes: it's strange because I'm not an enthusiastic runner, but if all runs were all like this I think I could take it up. I ran a different route, which always makes things more interesting and fun, especially when you get to run along a beach for a couple of miles.

YOUR TRAINING SESSION

AM

PM **Training session** CV – Run

Time trained

Session time

RPE /10

WORKOUT
Run – 6 miles
Actual distance: miles
Time: minutes
Average pace: m/m

Your notes:

TRAINING SESSION **WEEK 7** DAY 2

MY TRAINING SESSION

AM Rest

PM Training session Weights – Chest and back

Time trained 6.35–7.40 p.m.

Session time 1 hour 5 minutes

RPE 7/10

WORKOUT

Incline press
1 × 20 warm-up – with just Olympic bar
Set and Rep: 1. 10   2. 10   3. 10   4. 10   5. 10
Weight (kg):   40   50   90   90   90

Pull-ups
Regular: 2, 4, 6, 8, 10
Wide: 2, 4, 6, 8, 10
Close: 2, 4, 6, 8, 10
Mountain climbers: 2, 4, 6, 8, 10
Reverse: 2, 4, 6, 8, 10

Superset

	Bench press				Rope pulls			
Sets	1.	2.	3.	4.	1.	2.	3.	4
Reps	10	10	8	7	10	10	10	10
Weight (kg)	90	105	110	110	50	50	50	50

Morey squeeze (upper – cable)
Set and Rep: 1. 15   2. 10   3. 10
Weight (kg):   10   10   10

My notes: for today's session I added the new pull-ups, which I love. You can feel it hit your whole back and give you an all over pump for that area. I did a personal training session today, which only involved me power walking for one mile so I didn't note this on your training diary.

YOUR TRAINING SESSION

AM

PM Training session Weights – Chest and back

Time trained

Session time

RPE   /10

WORKOUT

Incline press
1 × 20 warm-up – with just Olympic bar
Set and Rep: 1.   2.   3.   4.   5.
Weight (kg):

Pull-ups
Regular: 2, 4, 6, 8, 10
Wide: 2, 4, 6, 8, 10
Close: 2, 4, 6, 8, 10
Mountain climbers: 2, 4, 6, 8, 10
Reverse: 2, 4, 6, 8, 10

Superset

	Bench press				Rope pulls			
Sets	1.	2.	3.	4.	1.	2.	3.	4.
Reps								
Weight (kg)								

Morey squeeze (upper – cable)
Set and Rep: 1.   2.   3.
Weight (kg):

Your notes:

TRAINING SESSION **WEEK 7** DAY 3

MY TRAINING SESSION

AM Rest

PM **Training session** CV – Run

Time trained 6.40–7.15 p.m.

Session time 35 minutes

RPE 8/10

WORKOUT
Run – 4 miles
Actual distance: 4.01 miles
Time: 32.00 minutes
Average pace: 8.00 m/m

My notes: I really didn't want to train today, so mentally I found the run more like RPE 10/10. By the end I was glad to have finished.

YOUR TRAINING SESSION

AM

PM **Training session** CV – Run

Time trained

Session time

RPE   /10

WORKOUT
Run – 4 miles
Actual distance: miles
Time: minutes
Average pace: m/m

Your notes:

TRAINING SESSION **WEEK 7** DAY 4

MY TRAINING SESSION

AM Rest

PM **Training session** Weights – Shoulders and arms

Time trained 8.00–9.25 p.m.

Session time 1 hour 25 minutes

RPE 6/10

YOUR TRAINING SESSION

AM

PM **Training session** Weights – Shoulders and arms

Time trained

Session time

RPE   /10

WORKOUT

Military press
1 × 20 warm-up – with just Olympic bar

Set and Rep:	1. 10	2. 10	3. 10	4. 10	5. 10
Weight (kg):	30	40	50	50	50

Upright rows (cable)

Set and Rep:	1. 10	2. 10	3. 10	4. 10
Weight (kg):	40	40	40	40

Reverse shrug

Set and Rep:	1. 10	2. 10	3. 10	4. 10
Weight (kg):	50	90	90	90

Bent-over lat raise – drop set

Set and Rep:	1. 10	2.1 0	3. 10	4. 10	5. 10	6. 10
Weight (lb):	40	20	40	20	40	20

Rope triceps press-down

Set and Rep:	1. 10	2. 10	3. 10
Weight (kg):	25	25	25

Supernated curl

Set and Rep:	1. 10	2. 10	3. 10
Weight (lb):	40	40	40

Abs cycle
½ sit-ups (1 set of the 3 types of sit-ups × 20 reps)
Reverse curls: 3 × 10
Leg levers: 3 × 10

My notes: I started well but it was a bit too late for me to train so I started to fade near the end hence only two arm exercises, but this was the only time I could train so it had to be then.

WORKOUT

Military press
1 × 20 warm-up – with just Olympic bar

Set and Rep:	1.	2.	3.	4.	5.
Weight (kg):					

Upright rows (cable)

Set and Rep:	1.	2.	3.	4.
Weight (kg):				

Reverse shrug

Set and Rep:	1.	2.	3.	4.
Weight (kg):				

Bent-over lat raise – drop set

Set and Rep:	1.	2.	3.	4.	5.	6.
Weight (kg):						

Rope triceps press-down

Set and Rep:	1.	2.	3.
Weight (kg):			

Supernated curl

Set and Rep:	1.	2.	3.
Weight (kg):			

Abs cycle
½ sit-ups (1 set of the 3 types of sit-ups × 20 reps)
Reverse curls: 3 ×
Leg levers: 3 ×

Your notes:

TRAINING SESSION **WEEK 7** DAY 5

MY TRAINING SESSION

AM Rest

PM Training session PT – Lower body

Time trained 56.00–6.35 p.m.

Session time 35 minutes

RPE 7/10

WORKOUT

No rest in between sets and reps on pull-ups, press-ups and sit-ups.

Squat jump: 4 × 15
Static lunge, right leg: 4 × 15
Static lunge, left leg: 4 × 15
Calf raise: 4 × 15
Jump over: 4 × 15
Frog hop: 4 × 15
Reverse Curls: 3 × 20
½ sit ups: 3 × 20
Full sit ups: 3 × 20
Heel taps: 3 × 20

My notes: This is always a great leg workout due to the plyometric training. Be careful not to put too much plyometric training into your own training as it can increase a risk of injury.

YOUR TRAINING SESSION

AM

PM Training session PT – Upper body

Time trained

Session time

RPE   /10

WORKOUT

Static jump: ×
Static lunge, right leg: ×
Static lunge, left leg: ×
Calf raise: ×
Jump over: ×
Frog hop: ×
Reverse Curls: ×
½ sit ups: ×
Full sit ups: ×
Heel taps: ×

Your notes:

TRAINING SESSION **WEEK 7** DAY 6

MY TRAINING SESSION

AM Rest

PM **Training session** Circuits

Time trained 7.30–8.05 p.m.

Session time 35 minutes

RPE 9/10

YOUR TRAINING SESSION

AM

PM **Training session** Circuits

Time trained

Session time

RPE /10

WORKOUT

Each station comprises a weighted exercise, then a mat exercise, then a body weight exercise. Complete all the exercises in station 1, then rest (if required) before moving onto the second station. Continue until you have completed all 10 stations. Each exercise lasts for 1 minute.

I used 20kg (just the Olympic bar) for the weighted exercises.

1. Military press – full sit-ups – squat thrusts
2. Squats – V sit-ups – alternate squat thrusts
3. Bent over rows – 1/2 sit-ups – star jumps
4. Upright rows – reverse curls – press-ups
5. Arm curls – plank – jumping oblique twists
6. Overhead triceps ext – reverse crunch – burpees
7. Wide grip bent over rows – crunch – wide squat thrusts
8. Static lunge right leg – heel taps – diamond press-ups
9. Static lunge left leg – dorsal raise – spotty dogs
10. Calf raise – leg levers – wide press-ups

My notes: My legs were aching too much to do any type of running or exercises. Go as fast as you can for each minute and you will get an amazing feeling at the end.

Your notes:

WEEK 7 TESTS

Front view of me at the end of week 7.

Back view of me at the end of week 7.

MY WEEKLY TESTS

Weight (kg):   79
Height (cm):   175.5
BMI: 25.6
RHR: 48
BP: 145/45
Fat %:   13.5

Measurements (cm)
Neck: 38.73
Chest: 104.77
Arm: R 37.46   L 37.46
Navel: 80.64
Hips: 83.82
Thighs: R 60.96   L 60.96
Calves: R 40   L 40

YOUR WEEKLY TESTS

Weight (kg):
Height (cm):
BMI:
RHR:
BP:
Fat %:

Measurements (cm)
Neck:
Chest:
Arm: R   L
Navel:
Hips:
Thighs: R   L
Calves: R   L

WEEK **EIGHT** NUTRITION PLAN **WEEK 8**

WEEK 8 OVERVIEW

Day	Breakfast	Lunch	Dinner
1	Fresh fruit and seeds	Sweet potato and bean salad	Mackerel and pine nut salad
2	Fruit porridge	Tuna and olive salad	Broccoli and chicken stir fry
3	Muesli with fresh fruit	Vegetable soup	Teriyaki burgers
4	Fruit smoothie 1	Beef salad pitta	Chilli prawns with almonds
5	Fresh fruit and seeds	Mackerel and potato salad	Mustard chicken
6	Omelette	Smoked salmon pitta	Garlic salmon with baked vegetables
7	Wheat biscuits or muesli with fruit	Tuna salad	Lamb casserole

SHOPPING LIST **WEEK 8**

CARBOHYDRATES
80g almonds
1 bag of brown rice
1 bag of couscous
400g kidney beans
240g of muesli
1 bag of pine nuts
125g new potatoes
400g pinto beans
560g porridge oats
12 potatoes
1 bag of sunflower seeds
1 bag of pumpkin seeds
8 sweet potatoes
8 wholemeal/brown pitta
  breads
Wheat biscuits

DAIRY AND NON-DAIRY ALTERNATIVES
12 eggs
20g feta/goat's cheese
50g soft goat's/low fat
  cream cheese
880ml skimmed/ soya/rice/
  oat milk
1.7kg soya yoghurt

FISH
8 anchovy fillets
4 whole mackerel, scaled/
  gutted
225g fresh mackerel
800g cooked prawns
4 salmon fillets
1 pack smoked salmon (for
  four people)
1.15kg tuna steaks
4 tinned tuna cans

MEAT
500g lean minced beef
400g cooked, roast beef
8 chicken breasts
400g lean ham

800g leg of lamb

FRUIT
4 apples
1 apricot
8 bananas
1 punnet of blackberries
1 punnet of blueberries
3 lemons
2 limes
2 mangos
1 melon
2 oranges
1 peach
1 large pineapple
1 punnet of raspberries

VEGETABLES
2 avocados
600g baby spinach
25g black olives
75g broccoli
250g cherry tomatoes
3 carrots
1 celery stick
1 courgette
½ cucumber
175g French beans
2 leeks
3 lettuces
50g mangetout
5 onions
2 parsnips
115g plum tomatoes
3 red onions
4 red peppers
23 tomatoes
100g rocket salad
1 shallot
10 spring onions

HERBS
Basil
2 bay leaves

Black pepper
Chives
Coriander
Cumin
Fresh ginger
1 garlic bulb
Parsley
2 red chillies
Rosemary

OTHER
Balsamic vinegar
Chicken stock
Chinese rice wine
Cold-pressed extra virgin
  olive oil
Corn flour
Dijon mustard
Light soy sauce
Peanut oil
60ml red wine
Sesame oil
Soy sauce
Brown sugar
400g tinned tomatoes
Tomato purée
Vegetable stock
White wine vinegar
Wholegrain mustard

SNACKS
Fruit
Wholegrain crispbread
  crackers
Flat breads
Small bowl of muesli
Yoghurt/soya yoghurt
Nuts (cashew, pine or
  occasionally mixed nuts)
Soya nuts
Seeds (pumpkin or sunflower)

FRUIT DRINKS
1 carton fruit juice

RECIPES **WEEK 8** DAY 1

BREAKFAST FRESH FRUIT AND SEEDS

See page 82

LUNCH SWEET POTATO AND BEAN SALAD

4 cooked sweet potatoes

4 eggs

2 avocados, stoned and peeled

400g tinned kidney beans

400g tinned pinto beans

Coriander, large handful chopped

250g cherry tomatoes, halved

1 small red onion, finely sliced

1 Preheat oven to 190°C (375°F).
2 Boil eggs for 6½ minutes, then place in cold water to cool slightly.
3 Cut the sweet potatoes into small chunks and drizzle with a tablespoon of olive oil and place into oven for 30–40 minutes.
4 Slice avocados and place in bowl with beans, sweet potatoes, onions, coriander and tomatoes.
5 Mix the olive oil, lime juice, chilli and cumin in a small bowl.
6 Once eggs have cooled but are still warm, peel off the shells and cut into quarters.
7 Toss the salad with the dressing, place the eggs on top and serve.

DINNER MACKEREL AND PINE NUT SALAD

4 whole mackerel, scaled and gutted

1 clove of garlic, peeled and sliced

4 tablespoon parsley, chopped

4 spring onions, trimmed and chopped

3 tablespoons pine nuts

1 lemon, zest of

Salad of your choice

1 Preheat the grill to high and cover the grill tray with tin foil.
2 Make two incisions in the side of each mackerel and fill with garlic and parsley and place on a tray.
3 Mix the spring onions, pine nuts and lemon zest in a small bowl and use to stuff the cavity of the mackerel.
4 Place fish under the hot grill and cook for 3–4 minutes on each side or until cooked.
5 Remove the mackerel from the grill and allow to cool for a few minutes. Serve with salad.

RECIPES **WEEK 8** DAY 2

BREAKFAST FRUIT PORRIDGE   *See page 81*

LUNCH TUNA AND OLIVE SALAD   *See page 81*

DINNER BROCCOLI AND CHICKEN STIR FRY

800g skinless chicken breasts, diced

1 head broccoli, broken into florets

1 tablespoon ginger, freshly grated

1 clove garlic, crushed

1 onion, quartered

1 red pepper, deseeded and sliced

2 tablespoons water

2 teaspoons Chinese rice wine

1 tablespoon soy sauce

2 teaspoons corn flour

1 teaspoon sesame oil

1 tablespoon peanut oil

Brown rice

1 Bring a small saucepan of water to the boil and blanch the broccoli for 2 minutes. Drain, and allow to cool.
2 In a cup, mix together the water, Chinese rice wine, soy sauce and corn flour and set aside.
3 Heat a wok or large frying pan over a medium heat.
4 Add sesame and peanut oil, and once smoking add the ginger and garlic and cook for a few seconds, stirring continuously.
5 Add the chicken and stir fry for 6–8 minutes, or until cooked. Remove from wok and set aside.
6 Boil the rice. Add the onion and red pepper to frying pan and stir fry for 5 minutes, or until vegetables begin to soften.
7 Next add the broccoli and corn flour, and stir until sauce has thickened.
8 Return chicken to the frying pan and heat through. Serve with brown rice.

Lunch for tomorrow:
VEGETABLE SOUP
Consider preparing your lunch in advance.

RECIPES **WEEK 8** DAY 3

BREAKFAST MUESLI WITH FRESH FRUIT

See page 80

LUNCH VEGETABLE SOUP

See page 100

DINNER TERIYAKI BURGERS

500g lean minced beef

2 tablespoons light soy sauce

1 tablespoon fresh ginger, peeled and grated

1 garlic clove, minced

¼ cup onions, chopped

Pinch of pepper

4 baking potatoes, sliced into wedges

Lettuce leaves

3 tomatoes, sliced

1 small red onion, sliced

20g goat's or mature cheese, 5g per person

1 Preheat oven to 190°C (373 F).
2 Boil the potato wedges until partially tender.
3 Place wedges on a baking tray and drizzle over extra virgin olive oil.
4 Cook in the oven until crisp and golden.
5 Combine all the ingredients for the burgers in a bowl.
6 Form into 4–8 patties and grill for 5 minutes one side then turn over.
7 Place the cheese on the uncooked side and cook for a further 5 minutes or until cheese has melted.

RECIPES **WEEK 8** DAY 4

BREAKFAST FRUIT SMOOTHIE 1   *See page 87*

LUNCH BEEF SALAD PITTA   *See page 101*

DINNER CHILLI PRAWNS WITH ALMONDS

1 red chilli, finely chopped

1 tablespoon olive oil

1 onion, chopped

2 garlic cloves, roughly chopped

8 tomatoes, roughly chopped

1 teaspoon ground cumin

100ml chicken stock

80g ground almonds

150ml soya/plain yoghurt

800g cooked peeled prawns

1 lime

Brown rice and vegetables of your choice

1 Heat the olive oil in a frying pan over a medium heat.
2 Add the garlic, chilli and onion and cook until soft.
3 Next add the tomatoes and ground cumin and cook for 10 minutes, stirring occasionally.
4 Add the stock to the mixture and blend in a food processor until smooth.
5 Pour the mixture into a large saucepan, adding the ground almonds, and stir over a low heat for 2 minutes.
6 Gently stir in the yoghurt.
7 Squeeze the juice from the lime and stir into sauce.
8 Increase the heat and simmer.
9 Add the prawns and heat for 2–3 minutes until warmed through.
10 Serve with brown rice and vegetables.

Lunch for tomorrow:
MACKEREL AND POTATO SALAD
Consider preparing the potatoes in advance (refrigerate overnight).

RECIPES **WEEK 8** DAY 5

BREAKFAST FRESH FRUIT
AND SEEDS

See page 82

LUNCH MACKEREL
AND POTATO SALAD

See page 134

DINNER MUSTARD CHICKEN

1 tablespoon olive oil

4 chicken breasts, fat removed

2 large oranges, peeled and cut into
segments (reserve the juice)

2 teaspoons cornflour

150ml soya/plain yoghurt

1 teaspoon wholegrain mustard

Parsley to garnish

Couscous, salad or vegetables of your choice

1. Heat the olive oil in a large frying pan and add the chicken breasts.
2. Cook over a medium to high heat for 5 minutes on each side, or until tender and the juices run clear.
3. Season with black pepper, then remove chicken from frying pan and cover with foil and keep warm.
4. Pour the orange juice into a bowl and stir in the corn flour to make a smooth paste.
5. Stir in yoghurt and mustard then pour into the frying pan. Bring to the boil over a low heat while stirring.
6. Add the orange segments to the frying pan and season to taste with pepper.
7. Stir in the juices from the chicken. Spoon the sauce on to four large plates and top with chicken.
8. Serve with salad or vegetables and couscous, and garnish with parsley.

RECIPES **WEEK 8** DAY 6

BREAKFAST OMELETTE   *See page 88*

LUNCH SMOKED SALMON PITTA   *See page 80*

DINNER GARLIC SALMON WITH BAKED VEGETABLES

2 leeks, washed, trimmed and sliced

500g baby spinach leaves

4 × 100g salmon fillets

1 tablespoon olive oil

2 garlic cloves, peeled and finely chopped

1 tablespoon fresh ginger, grated

1 lemon, juice of

Coriander to garnish

Couscous

1 Preheat the oven to 200°C (400°F).
2 Gently boil or steam the leeks for 5 minutes.
3 Arrange the spinach leaves in a baking tray, then add the leeks and place salmon on top.
4 Mix together the olive oil, garlic and ginger in a small bowl and brush mixture over the salmon using pastry brush.
5 Pour over the lemon juice, place in the oven and cook for 10 minutes.
6 Boil and cook couscous.
7 Remove from oven and leave to cool for a few minutes.
8 Serve with couscous and garnish with fresh coriander.

RECIPES **WEEK 8** DAY 7

BREAKFAST WHEAT BISCUITS OR
MUESLI WITH FRUIT

See page 84

LUNCH TUNA SALAD

See page 131

DINNER LAMB CASSEROLE

800g lean lamb leg, diced

2 tablespoons olive oil

1 onion, finely chopped

1 carrot, finely chopped

1 celery stick, finely chopped

2 cloves garlic, crushed

60ml red wine

2 tablespoons tomato purée

450ml chicken stock

1 bay leaf

2 sprigs rosemary

2 parsnips, peeled and chopped

2 tablespoons parsley

New potatoes

1 Preheat oven to 180°C (350°F).
2 Heat a large saucepan over a high heat.
3 Coat lamb with olive oil and cook in small batches for 5 minutes or until browned.
4 Remove from pan and set aside.
5 Add the onion, carrot, celery to the pan and cook for 5 minutes, or until soft.
6 Next, return lamb to pan adding the garlic, red wine and tomato purée and cook for a further 5 minutes.
7 Add the chicken stock, bay leaf, rosemary and enough water to ensure lamb is covered.
8 Cover with lid and bake in the oven for 1 hour.
9 Add the parsnips and cook for a further 40 minutes.
10 Serve with potatoes and sprinkle with parsley.

TRAINING DIARY **WEEK 8**

WEEK 8 OVERVIEW
Day 1: PT- Upper body
Day 2: Weights – Chest and back
Day 3: Weights – Legs
Day 4: Rest
Day 5: Circuits; Weights – Shoulders and arms
Day 6: CV – Cycle
Day 7: Test day
Any day: Myo stretch

MY DIARY

Day 1 (Monday)
Went to work as normal, had a massage to help my posture.
Tiredness 2
Stress 3
Sleep 6 hours 45 minutes

Day 2 (Tuesday)
I was looking forward to training as I'm trying to beat my personal best on the bench press.
Tiredness 2
Stress 2
Sleep 7 hours

Day 3 (Wednesday)
My upper body is slightly sore all over, which showed me I had a good session last night. Didn't manage to have dinner tonight as I was running late with work and had to meet up with some friends, but I did manage to get a snack instead, as well as fit in my training session.
Tiredness 3
Stress 1
Sleep 6 hours

Day 4 (Thursday)
I'm renovating my gym today, ready for my clients next week. My legs and glutes are now aching from yesterday's session, which is fantastic. Still got a little bit of family stress, but I'm using the same rules that are in the health chapter.
Tiredness 3
Stress 3
Sleep 8 hours 30 minutes

Day 5 (Friday)
I've been feeling rather fat recently due to not eating dinner a couple of days ago and having dinner at Alison's last night. I did circuit training to help burn some excess fat.
Tiredness 2
Stress 1
Sleep 6 hours 45 minutes

Day 6 (Saturday)
I cycled to Poole from my house. For the first time in what seems like a lifetime it was extremely hard. There were so many points in the cycle I wanted to quit, but mentally I was fighting it all the way. When I got there I was so relieved and proud of knowing I can do anything if I set my mind to it.
Tiredness 3
Stress 1
Sleep 8 hours

Day 7 (Sunday)
Test day today, so I think I was wrong to cycle yesterday as I was still feeling tired from it, but I gave the test 100% and it paid off as once again my results were getting better.
Tiredness 4
Stress 3
Sleep 4 hours 30 minutes

TRAINING SESSION **WEEK 8** DAY 1

MY TRAINING SESSION

AM Rest

PM Training session PT – Upper body

Time trained 5.55–6.40 p.m.

Session time 45 minutes

RPE 7/10

WORKOUT

No rest in between sets and reps on pull-ups, press-ups and sit-ups.

Chest and abs cycle × 20
Regular press-ups: × 10
½ sit-ups: × 10
Diamond press-ups: × 10
Leg levers: × 10
Wide push-ups: × 10
Crunches: × 10
Total press-ups: 600
Total sit-ups: 600

Arm haulers : 3 × 50

My notes: Got back into the gym today after having a day off. It felt as if I had so much energy that I could just keep going – it's just amazing what a day off can do.

YOUR TRAINING SESSION

AM

PM   Training session PT – Upper body

Time trained

Session time

RPE   /10

WORKOUT

Chest and abs cycle   ×
Regular press-ups: ×
½ sit-ups: ×
Diamond press-ups: ×
Leg levers: ×
Wide push-ups: ×
Crunches: ×
Total press-ups:
Total sit-ups:

Arm haulers :   *3* ×

Your notes:

TRAINING SESSION **WEEK 8** DAY 2

MY TRAINING SESSION

AM Rest

PM **Training session** Weights – Chest and back

Time trained 5.40–7.00 p.m.

Session time 1 hour 20 minutes

RPE 7/10

WORKOUT

Bench press
1 × 20 warm-up – with just Olympic bar
Set and Rep: 1. 20 2. 15 3. 10 4. 10 5. 6 6. 6
Weight (kg): 40 50 80 90 110 112.5

Deadlift
1 × 20 warm-up – with just Olympic bar
Set and Rep: 1. 10 2. 10 3. 10 4. 10
Weight (kg): 90 110 120 120

Superset

	Straight arm pull-overs			Morey squeeze (lower – cable)		
Set and Rep	1. 10	2. 10	3. 10	1. 10	2. 10	3. 10
Weight (kg)	52.5	52.5	52.5	10	10	10

T-bar row
Set and Rep: 1. 10 2. 10 3. 10 4. 10
Weight (kg): 35 45 50 50

My notes: As I felt I had so much energy, I went heavy on my bench press and deadlifts. I managed to lift my heaviest weight for years.

YOUR TRAINING SESSION

AM

PM **Training session** Weights – Chest and back

Time trained

Session time

RPE /10

WORKOUT

Bench press
1 × 20 warm-up – with just Olympic bar
Set and Rep: 1. 2. 3. 4. 5. 6.
Weight (kg):

Deadlift
1 × 20 warm-up – with just Olympic bar
Set and Rep: 1. 2. 3. 4.
Weight (kg):

Superset

	Straight arm pull-overs			Morey squeeze (lower – cable)		
Set and Rep	1.	2.	3.	1.	2.	3.
Weight (kg)						

T-bar row
Set and Rep: 1. 2. 3. 4.
Weight (kg):

Your notes:

TRAINING SESSION **WEEK 8** DAY 3

MY TRAINING SESSION

AM Rest

PM **Training session** Weights – Legs

Time trained 6.00–7.10 p.m.

Session time 1 hour 10 minutes

RPE 6/10

WORKOUT

Static lunges (dumbbells)
1 × 20 warm-up (no weight)
Set and Rep: 1. 16   2. 16   3. 16   4. 16
Weight (lb):   55   55   55   55

Sissy squats
Set and Rep: 1. 10   2. 10   3. 10   4. 10

Stiff leg deadlifts
Set and Rep: 1. 12   2. 12   3. 12   4. 12
Weight (kg):   75   75   75   75

Squats
1 × 20 warm-up – with just Olympic bar
Set and Rep: 1. 16 2. 16 3. 12 4. 12   5. 12 6. 16
Weight (kg):   60   80   110   110   110   60

Calf raises
Set and Rep: 1. 20   2. 20   3. 20   4. 20   5. 15
Weight (kg):   90   110   110   110   110

My notes: I could feel my whole back from yesterday's deadlifts, and even my hamstrings. Squats – on the 6th set I chose to put the weight down to get as low as possible and the most out of my quads. I'm starting to have a love/hate relationship with squats, mainly because it hurts so much, but I'm enjoying the feeling.

YOUR TRAINING SESSION

AM

PM   **Training session** Weights – Legs

Time trained

Session time

RPE   /10

WORKOUT

Static lunges (dumbbells)
1 × 20 warm-up (no weight)
Set and Rep: 1.   2.   3.   4.
Weight (lb):

Sissy squats
Set and Rep: 1.   2.   3.   4.

Stiff leg deadlifts
Set and Rep: 1.   2.   3.   4.
Weight (kg):

Squats
1 × 20 warm-up – with just Olympic bar
Set and Rep: 1.   2.   3.   4.   5.   6.
Weight (kg):

Calf raises
Set and Rep: 1.   2.   3.   4.
Weight (kg):

Your notes:

TRAINING SESSION **WEEK 8** DAY 5

MY TRAINING SESSION

AM Rest

PM Training session Weights – Shoulders and arms

Time trained 10.00–11.15 a.m.

Session time 1 hour 15 minutes

RPE 7/10

PM Training session Circuits

Time trained 6.00–7.10 p.m.

Session time 1 hour 10 minutes

RPE 7/10

YOUR TRAINING SESSION

AM

PM Training session CV – Shoulders and arms

Time trained

Session time

RPE /10

PM Training session Circuits

Time trained

Session time

RPE /10

WORKOUT

Military press
1 × 20 warm-up – with just Olympic bar

Set and Rep:	1. 10	2. 10	3. 10	4. 10	5. 8
Weight (kg):	30	40	50	50	55

Reverse shrug

Set and Rep:	1. 10	2. 10	3. 10	4. 10
Weight (kg):	50	90	90	100

Lat raise

Set and Rep:	1. 10	2. 10	3. 10
Weight (lb):	35	35	40

Overhead triceps extension

Set and Rep:	1. 10	2. 10	3. 10	4. 7
Weight (kg):	25	30	35	40

WORKOUT

Military press
1 × 20 warm-up – with just Olympic bar

Set and Rep:	1.	2.	3.	4.	5.
Weight (kg):					

Reverse shrug

Set and Rep:	1.	2.	3.	4.
Weight (kg):				

Lat raise

Set and Rep:	1.	2.	3.
Weight (kg):			

Overhead triceps extension

Set and Rep:	1.	2.	3.	4.
Weight (kg):				

Concentrated curl

Set and Rep:	1. 10	2. 10	3. 8	4. 7
Weight (lb):	40	40	40	40

Superset

	Preacher curl			Single arm pull-down		
Set and Rep	1. 10	2. 10	3. 10	1. 20	2. 20	3. 15
Weight (kg)	30	30	30	5	5	7.5

WORKOUT

For the circuits session, complete cycle 1 first, then cycle 2, and finally cycle 3.

Cycle 1

Weight used for all exercises: 13kg. Each exercise lasts for 1 minute 30 seconds.

1. Lunge jumps   1. Deadlifts   1. Bent-over lat raise
2. Squat jumps   2. Chest press 2. Incline press
3. Jump overs   3. Lat raise   3. Calf raises

Cycle 2

Weight bar: 30kg; dumbbells (DB): 7kg.
Do 30 reps for all exercises.

1. Jump overs
2. V-sit-ups
3. Lat raises (DB)
4. Bent-over lat raise
5. Deadlift (bar)
6. Squat bosu
7. Dips
8. Wide squats thrusts
9. Leg levers
10. Arm curl (bar)
11. Lunge bosu – per leg
12. Arm haulers
13. Walking hands on step

Cycle 3

Do 30 reps for all exercises.

1. Straight punches
2. ½ sit-ups
3. Alternate punches
4. Oblique side crunches
5. Upper cut punches
6. V-sit-ups
7. Wide punches
8. Reverse curls

Finish with a 2-minute plank

Concentrated curl

Set and Rep:	1.	2.	3.	4.
Weight (kg):				

Superset

	Preacher curl			Single arm pull-down		
Set and Rep:	1.	2.	3.	1.	2.	3.
Weight (kg):						

WORKOUT

Your notes:

TRAINING SESSION **WEEK 8** DAY 6

MY TRAINING SESSION

AM Rest

PM **Training session** CV– Cycle

Time trained 6.50–8.10 p.m.

Session time 1 hour 20 minutes

RPE 10/10

WORKOUT
Cycle – 20 miles
Actual distance: 20.5 miles

My notes: I cycled from New Milton to Poole to see my friend. I did this cycle about three years ago, but I don't remember it being this hard. The weather was extreme due to the high winds. At one point along the sea front it felt as if I wasn't moving at all. There were four or five times when I had to coast because my legs couldn't take it. When I got to my friend's I then had to walk about a mile to meet some other friends, so I felt rather knackered by the end of the day.

YOUR TRAINING SESSION

AM

PM **Training session** Cycle

Time trained

Session time

RPE   /10

WORKOUT
Cycle – 20 miles
Actual distance: miles

Your notes:

Front and back views of me
at the end of week 8.

WEEK 8 HEALTH CHECK

MY RESULTS

Statistics	Weight (kg): 78.5
	Height (cm): 175.5
Health tests	BMI: 25.5
	RHR: 45
	BP: 138/44
	Fat (%): 13.2
	Glucose: 5.1
	Cholesterol: 3.9
	Lung function: 670
Measurements (cm)	Neck: 38.73
	Chest: 106.04
	Arms: R: 37.46 L: 37.46
	Navel: 79.37
	Hips: 83.18
	Thighs: R: 61.59 L: 61.59
	Calves: R: 40 L: 40
Calliper test (mm)	Biceps: 3
	Triceps: 6
	Waist: 9
	Subscapularis: 9
	Total: 27
	Calliper fat (%): 11.9
Fitness tests	Bleep test (level): 12.5
Maximum reps in one minute	Push-ups: 80
	½ sit-ups: 99
	Squats: 78
	Dips: 90
	Max pull-ups: 35
One rep maximum weight training (kg)	Squats: 132.5
	Bench press: 120
	Military press: 64
	Deadlifts: 132.5

YOUR RESULTS

Statistics	Weight (kg):
	Height (cm):
Health tests	BMI:
	RHR:
	BP: /
	Fat (%):
	Glucose:
	Cholesterol:
	Lung function:
Measurements (cm)	Neck:
	Chest:
	Arms: R: L:
	Navel:
	Hips:
	Thighs: R: L:
	Calves: R: L:
Calliper test (mm)	Biceps:
	Triceps:
	Waist:
	Subscapularis:
	Total:
	Calliper fat (%):
Fitness tests	Bleep test (level):
Maximum reps in one minute	Push-ups:
	½ sit-ups:
	Squats:
	Dips:
	Max pull-ups:
One rep maximum weight training (kg)	Squats:
	Bench press:
	Military press:
	Deadlifts:

WEEK NINE NUTRITION PLAN **WEEK 9**

WEEK 9 OVERVIEW

Day	Breakfast	Lunch	Dinner
1	Fresh fruit and seeds	Beetroot salad	Coconut monkfish
2	Fruit smoothie 2	Yellow split pea soup	Chicken with coriander
3	Muesli with fresh fruit	Egg salad	Cajun fish
4	Wheat biscuits or muesli with fruit	Salmon salad	Thai beef salad
5	Fruit porridge	Tuna salad	Spicy tomato chicken
6	Omelette	Butternut squash and coriander soup	Salmon with asparagus
7	Fruit salad	Chicken salad pitta	Ginger turkey curry

SHOPPING LIST **WEEK 9**

CARBOHYDRATES
1 bag of brown rice
1 bag of couscous
260g of muesli
560g porridge oats
1 bag of sunflower seeds
1 bag of pumpkin seeds
5 sweet potatoes
4 wholemeal/brown pitta
   breads
225g yellow split peas
1 bag of wild rice
Wheat biscuits

DAIRY AND NON-DAIRY ALTERNATIVES
12 eggs
2105ml skimmed/soya/rice/
   oat milk
2kg soya yoghurt

FISH
6 anchovy fillets
450g monkfish tails
225g raw peeled prawns
4 poached salmon fillets
200g × 4 salmon steaks
4 tins of tuna
800g white fish of your
   choice

MEAT
800g rump beef steak
500g boneless chicken
   breasts
8 chicken breasts
400g lean ham
400g turkey breast

FRUIT
8 apples
2 apricots

6 bananas
1 punnet of blackberries
1 punnet of blueberries
4 lemons
2 limes
1 melon
2 oranges
2 peaches
1 large pineapple
1 punnet of raspberries

VEGETABLES
16 asparagus spears
1 avocado
1 baby gem lettuce
350g baby spinach
150g bean sprouts
4 cooked beetroots
1.4kg butternut squash
650g cherry tomatoes
5 carrots
2 celery sticks
1 courgette
1½ cucumbers
3 lettuce
50g mangetout
4 onions
3 red onions
4 red peppers
5 red tomatoes
100g rocket salad
5 shallots
13 spring onions
5 yellow peppers

HERBS
Chilli powder
Chives
Coriander
Ground coriander
Cumin
Curry powder

Fresh ginger
1 garlic bulb
1 green chilli
Mint
Nutmeg
Paprika
Parsley
1 red chilli
Rosemary
Turmeric

OTHER
Balsamic vinegar
Chicken stock
Cider vinegar
150ml coconut milk
Cold-pressed extra virgin
   olive oil
Corn flour
Dijon mustard
Fish sauce
Honey
115ml lemon juice
8 wooden skewers
Soy sauce
Tomato purée
Vegetable stock
Worcestershire sauce

SNACKS
Fruit
Wholegrain crispbread
   crackers
Flat breads
Small bowl of muesli
Yoghurt/soya yoghurt
Nuts (cashew, pine or
   occasionally mixed nuts)
Soya nuts
Seeds (pumpkin or sunflower)

FRUIT DRINKS
1 carton fruit juice

RECIPES **WEEK 9** DAY 1

BREAKFAST FRESH FRUIT
AND SEEDS

See page 82

LUNCH BEETROOT SALAD

See page 97

DINNER COCONUT MONKFISH

450g monkfish tails, cut into chunks

225g raw peeled prawns

1 red pepper, chunks to go on to skewers

1 yellow pepper, chunks to go on to skewers

1 red onion, chunks to go on to skewers

Salad leaves

Couscous

For the marinade:

1 teaspoon olive oil

½ small onion, finely grated

1 teaspoon fresh ginger, grated

150ml canned coconut milk

2 tablespoons fresh coriander, chopped

1 To make the marinade, heat the olive oil in a large saucepan and fry the onion and ginger for 5 minutes, or until just soft (not browned).

2 Add the coconut milk to the saucepan and bring to the boil.

3 Boil rapidly for 5 minutes then remove from heat and allow to cool completely.

4 Once cold, stir the coriander into the coconut milk and pour into a shallow dish.

5 Gently stir in monkfish and prawns into the coconut mixture and cover.

6 Leave to marinate in the fridge for 1–4 hours.

7 Preheat grill to medium.

8 Thread the fish and prawns on to skewers with the red onion and peppers.

9 Cook the skewers under the preheated grill for 10–15 minutes, turning frequently.

10 Garnish with toasted desiccated coconut and serve on a bed of salad and couscous.

Lunch for tomorrow:
YELLOW SPLIT PEA SOUP
Pre-soak the yellow split peas overnight in cold water.

RECIPES **WEEK 9** DAY 2

BREAKFAST FRUIT SMOOTHIE 2   *See page 152*

LUNCH YELLOW SPLIT PEA SOUP

225g yellow split peas (pre-soak for 12 hours overnight in cold water)

1.5 litres of vegetable stock

1 onion, peeled and sliced

1 sweet potato, peeled and chopped

3 carrots, trimmed, peeled and sliced

Fresh mint

Fresh baby spinach leaves, 4 handfuls

1 Drain water from the split peas.
2 Bring vegetable stock to the boil in a large saucepan and add split peas.
3 Simmer for 25 minutes, removing any scum on the surface.
4 Add all other vegetables to the saucepan and simmer for a further 15–20 minutes, or until vegetables are tender. Remove from heat and allow to cool.
5 Blend soup with food processor or blender.
6 Reheat soup and add the spinach. Serve with a mint garnish.

DINNER CHICKEN WITH CORIANDER

1 tablespoon olive oil

4 skinless, boneless chicken breasts 115g each, fat removed

1 teaspoon corn flour

1 tablespoon water

100ml soya/plain yoghurt

175ml chicken stock

2 tablespoons lime juice

2 garlic cloves, finely chopped

1 tomato, peeled, deseeded and chopped

1 shallot, finely chopped

Fresh coriander, 1 bunch chopped

Salad of your choice

1 Heat the olive oil in a large frying pan, then add the chicken and cook over medium heat for 5 minutes each side or until cooked.
2 Remove chicken from frying pan and keep warm.
3 Mix the corn flour and water until smooth. Stir in the yoghurt.
4 Pour the chicken stock and lime juice into frying pan and add the garlic and shallot.
5 Reduce the heat and simmer for 1 minute, then add the tomato and stir into mixture.
6 Cook and stir constantly for 1–2 minutes. Do not let the mixture boil.
7 Stir in the fresh coriander.
8 Serve the chicken with the salad, pour sauce over and garnish with fresh coriander.

Lunch for tomorrow:
EGG SALAD
Consider boiling eggs in advance (refrigerate overnight).

RECIPES **WEEK 9** DAY 3

BREAKFAST MUESLI WITH FRESH FRUIT

See page 80

LUNCH EGG SALAD

See page 116

DINNER CAJUN FISH

225ml soya/skimmed milk

800g white fish fillets (snapper, whiting, flathead etc.)

2 tablespoons olive oil

400g soya/plain yoghurt

½ cucumber, finely diced

Salad of your choice

Spices:

1 tablespoon paprika

2 teaspoons ground cumin

1 teaspoon chilli powder

1 Preheat oven to 200°C (400°F).
2 Line a baking tray with baking paper.
3 Pour the milk into a small bowl. In a separate bowl mix the ground spices.
4 Dip the fish fillets into the milk then roll in the mixed spices.
5 Heat the olive oil in a large frying pan over a high heat and fry the fish quickly in batches, for 2 minutes each side, or until golden. Be careful not overcrowd the pan, as the fish will stew.
6 Place the fish fillets on the baking tray and bake for 5 minutes.
7 Mix soya/plain yoghurt and cucumber to make the dressing.
8 Serve the fish with salad and pour over the yoghurt dressing.

RECIPES **WEEK 9** DAY 4

BREAKFAST WHEAT BISCUITS OR MUESLI WITH FRUIT

See page 84

LUNCH SALMON SALAD

See page 118

DINNER THAI BEEF SALAD

800g lean rump steak

1 tablespoon olive oil

For the salad:

100g spinach leaves

1 red pepper, deseeded and finely sliced

150g bean sprouts

4 spring onions, finely sliced

125g fresh coriander

2 tablespoons mint, chopped

For the dressing:

2 tablespoons lime juice

1 tablespoon fish sauce

1 tablespoon soy sauce

1 clove garlic, crushed

1 red chilli, deseeded and chopped

1 Preheat the grill to high.
2 Brush the steak with olive oil and cook for 3–4 minutes each side, or cook to your liking.
3 Remove from the heat and cover steak with tin foil and leave to rest for 5 minutes.
4 Meanwhile, mix all the dressing ingredients in a small bowl.
5 Slice the steak across the grain into thin strips. Place the beef and remaining ingredients in a large bowl.
6 Pour dressing over the salad, gently toss and serve.

**Lunch for tomorrow:
TUNA SALAD**
Consider preparing sweet potatoes for your lunch in advance.

RECIPES **WEEK 9** DAY 5

BREAKFAST FRUIT PORRIDGE

See page 81

LUNCH TUNA SALAD

See page 131

DINNER SPICY TOMATO CHICKEN

500g boneless chicken breasts, diced

3 tablespoons tomato purée

2 tablespoons clear honey

2 tablespoons Worcestershire sauce

1 tablespoon rosemary, chopped

250g cherry tomatoes

8 wooden skewers

Salad of your choice

1 Mix the tomato purée, honey, Worcestershire sauce and rosemary together in a bowl.
2 Add the diced chicken and coat evenly.
3 Preheat the grill to medium.
4 Thread the chicken and the cherry tomatoes on to the wooden skewers and place them on grill rack.
5 Spoon the honey mixture over the chicken skewers and grill for 8–10 minutes, turning occasionally until chicken is cooked through.
6 Serve with a salad.

RECIPES **WEEK 9** DAY 6

BREAKFAST OMELETTE   *See page 88*

LUNCH BUTTERNUT SQUASH   *See page 88*
AND CORIANDER SOUP

DINNER SALMON WITH ASPARAGUS

400g butternut squash, peeled
and cut into thick slices

1 tablespoon olive oil

4 × 200g salmon fillets

16 asparagus spears

For the relish:

Fresh parsley, 1 bunch

6 anchovy fillets

2 lemons, grated zest

115ml lemon juice

60ml olive oil

1 To make relish, place all the relish ingredients except olive oil in a food processor and lightly process.
2 Add olive oil to form a thick paste.
3 Preheat oven to 180°C (350°F).
4 Place the butternut squash in a bowl and coat with half the amount of olive oil.
5 Transfer to baking dish and cook for 20 minutes or until soft.
6 Meanwhile, turn grill to high and lightly brush the salmon with the remaining olive oil.
7 Place salmon in grill and cook for 4 minutes on each side.
8 Remove from heat, cover and set aside.
9 Bring a saucepan of water to the boil, add the asparagus and blanch for 2 minutes, then drain.
10 Arrange the salmon, asparagus and butternut squash slices on a serving plate and serve.

RECIPES **WEEK 9** DAY 7

BREAKFAST FRUIT SALAD
See page 85

LUNCH CHICKEN SALAD PITTA
See page 120

DINNER GINGER TURKEY CURRY

400g turkey fillet

½ tablespoon olive oil

1 onion, sliced

1 green chilli, finely sliced

12cm ginger, peeled and sliced

1 clove garlic, peeled and chopped

3 teaspoons curry powder

300ml chicken or vegetable stock

300g brown or wild rice

Coriander, big bunch

5 tablespoons soya/plain yoghurt

1 Heat the olive oil and add the onion, ginger, chilli and garlic. Cook on medium heat for 10 minutes.
2 Slice the turkey into small pieces, add to the pan with curry powder and cook for 5 minutes.
3 Add the stock, bring to the boil and simmer for 15 minutes.
4 Cook the rice on a medium heat for 15–20 minutes or until cooked.
5 Stir the yoghurt and chopped coriander through the turkey curry and serve with the rice.

Lunch for tomorrow:
BUTTERNUT SQUASH AND CORIANDER SOUP
Consider preparing in advance (refrigerate overnight).

TRAINING DIARY **WEEK 9**

WEEK 9 OVERVIEW
Day 1: Weights – Chest and back
Day 2: CV – Run
Day 3: Weights – Shoulders and arms
Day 4: CV – Run; Weights – Legs
Day 5: Weights – Chest and back;
      PT – Upper body
Day 6: CV – Walk
Day 7: Rest
Any day: Myo stretch

MY DIARY

Day 1 (Monday)
I had the intention of training this morning, but I didn't manage to get up in time. I decided to train later on today. By the time I got into the gym I wasn't feeling it, but as the session went on I felt as though I had a new lease of life.
Tiredness 3
Stress 2
Sleep 7 hours 45 minutes

Day 2 (Tuesday)
I had to do some running around today, which involved taking my family to the airport doing and some work.
Tiredness 4
Stress 2
Sleep 8 hours 30 minutes

Day 3 (Wednesday)
Day off today. I am finding the nutrition easy on the whole, but today after training I had a lovely dinner with Alison and a surprise dessert of dairy-free ice cream (ice cream is my Achilles heel when it comes to naughty food).
Tiredness 3
Stress 2
Sleep 8 hours

Day 4 (Thursday)
I loved today's session in the gym, but I don't know why as I pushed my legs really hard. I then had a massage to help release my legs afterwards so I didn't feel them too much the next day.
Tiredness 2
Stress 2
Sleep 7 hours 45 minutes

Day 5 (Friday)
Another hard day in the gym, and I'm now feeling as though it's time to give my body time off for a couple of days so that when I come back I will be stronger than ever.
Tiredness 2
Stress 2
Sleep 6 hours

Day 6 (Saturday)
I went to the Isle of Purbecks for a 15-mile walk with a close friend of mine. I just love this type of training, it really gets you fit with all those hills.
Tiredness 2
Stress 0
Sleep 6 hours

Day 7 (Sunday)
A well-earned day off today. My body is aching from yesterday's walk. I managed to have a myo massage which made my muscles feel in great shape.
Tiredness 3
Stress 2
Sleep 5 hours

TRAINING SESSION **WEEK 9** DAY 1

MY TRAINING SESSION

AM Rest

PM **Training session** Weights – Chest and back

Time trained 6.30–8.00 p.m.

Session time 1 hour 30 minutes

RPE 5/10

WORKOUT

Incline press
1 × 20 warm-up – with just Olympic bar
Set and Rep: 1. 15 2. 15 3. 10 4. 10 5. 10 6. 6
Weight (kg): 40   70   90   90   100   100

Superset

	Pec fly				Low pull (cable)			
Sets	1.	2.	3.	4.	1.	2.	3.	4
Reps	10	10	10	10	10	10	10	10
Weight (kg)	52.5	52.5	52.5	52.5	60	80	80	80

Pull-ups:
Regular: 2, 4, 6, 8, 10
Close: 2, 4, 6, 8, 10
Wide: 2, 4, 6, 8, 10
Reverse: 2, 4, 6, 8, 10
Mountain climbers: 2, 4, 6, 8, 10

Morey squeeze (upper – cable) – drop set
Set and Rep: 1. 10 1. 10 2. 10 2. 10 3. 10 3. 10
Weight (lb): 25   15   25   15   25   15

Rope pulls
Set and Rep: 1. 10 2. 10 3. 10 4. 10
Weight (kg): 15   17.5   17.5   17.5

YOUR TRAINING SESSION

AM

PM **Training session** Weights – Chest and back

Time trained

Session time

RPE   /10

WORKOUT

Incline press
1 × 20 warm-up – with just Olympic bar
Set and Rep: 1.   2.   3.   4.   5.   6.
Weight (kg):

Superset

	Pec fly				Low pull (cable)			
Sets	1.	2.	3.	4.	1.	2.	3.	4.
Reps								
Weight (kg)								

Pull-ups:
Regular:
Close:
Wide:
Reverse:
Mountain climbers:

Morey squeeze (upper – cable) – drop set
Set and Rep: 1.   2.   3.   1.   2.   3.
Weight (kg):

Rope pulls
Set and Rep: 1.   2.   3.   4.
Weight (kg):

½ sit-ups × 100

My notes: I did all 100 ½ sit-ups in one hit. Mentally this was difficult before I even started. As I got into the session, I got into the weights. This was quite a long and slow session, which enabled me to lift my heaviest weights on the incline press.

½ sit-ups ×

Your notes:

TRAINING SESSION **WEEK 9** DAY 2

MY TRAINING SESSION

AM Rest

PM **Training session** CV – Run

Time trained 5.00–6.05 p.m.

Session time 1 hour 5 minutes

RPE 7/10

WORKOUT
Run – 8 miles
Actual distance: 8.00 miles
Time: 1 hour 02 minutes
Average Pace: 7.45 m/m

My notes: the weather was raining and windy, which I quite enjoyed. The wind was with me on the way out and against me on the way back. I felt really strong until I got to around 5 miles, then I had a lull for around 0.5 miles. I managed to get through that and then it was plain sailing.

YOUR TRAINING SESSION

AM

PM **Training session** CV – Run

Time trained

Session time

RPE /10

WORKOUT
Run – 8 miles
Actual distance: miles
Time: minutes
Average Pace: m/m

Your notes:

TRAINING SESSION **WEEK 9** DAY 3

MY TRAINING SESSION

AM Rest

PM **Training session** Weights – Shoulders and arms

Time trained 1.50–3.00 p.m.

Session time 1 hour 10 minutes

RPE 8/10

WORKOUT
Military press
1 × 20 warm-up – with just Olympic bar

Set and Rep:	1. 10	2. 10	3. 8	4. 6	5. 6
Weight (kg):	30	50	55	55	55

Upright rows
Set and Rep:	1. 9	2. 8	3. 7	4. 8
Weight (kg):	55	55	55	55

Arm curl (Olympic bar)
Set and Rep:	1. 7	2. 6	3. 6	4. 6
Weight (kg):	50	50	50	50

Lat raise (cable)
Set and Rep:	1. 10	2. 10	3. 10
Weight (kg):	5	5	5

Bent-over lat raise (drop set)
Set and Rep:	1. 10	2. 10	3. 10	4. 10	5. 10	6. 10
Weight (lb):	40	20	40	20	40	20

Single arm pull-downs (cable)
Set and Rep:	1. 10	2. 10	3. 9
Weight (kg):	10	10	10

YOUR TRAINING SESSION

AM

PM **Training session** Weights – Shoulders and arms

Time trained

Session time

RPE   /10

WORKOUT
Military press
1 × 20 warm-up – with just Olympic bar

Set and Rep:	1.	2.	3.	4.	5.
Weight (kg):					

Upright rows
Set and Rep:	1.	2.	3.	4.
Weight (kg):				

Arm curl (Olympic bar)
Set and Rep:	1.	2.	3.	4.
Weight (kg):				

Lat raise (cable)
Set and Rep:	1.	2.	3.
Weight (kg):			

Bent-over lat raise (drop set)
Set and Rep:	1.	2.	3.	4.	5.	6.
Weight (kg):						

Single arm pull-downs (cable)
Set and Rep:	1.	2.	3.
Weight (kg):			

Rope triceps press-down
Set and Rep: 1. 10   2. 10   3. 9
Weight (kg):   27.5   27.5   27.5

Supernated curl
(drop set – no rest from 1st to 5th set)
Set and Rep: 1. 12   2. 10   3. 12   4. 15   5. 15
Weight (lb):   55   35   20   10   5

My notes: all of the sets were done to failure with the supernated curl. Amazing session for my arms, but for some reason my shoulders couldn't give me any more.

Rope triceps press-down
Set and Rep: 1.   2.   3.
Weight (kg):

Supernated curl
(drop set – no rest from 1st to 5th set)
Set and Rep: 1.   2.   3.   4.   5.
Weight (kg):

Your notes:

TRAINING SESSION **WEEK 9** DAY 4

MY TRAINING SESSION

AM Rest

PM Training session CV – Run

Time trained 5.40–6.02 p.m.

Session time 22 minutes

RPE 9/10

PM Training session Weights – Legs

Time trained 6.05–7.24 p.m.

Session time 1 hour 19 minutes

RPE 8/10

YOUR TRAINING SESSION

AM

PM Training session CV – Run

Time trained

Session time

RPE   /10

PM Training session Legs

Time trained

Session time

RPE   /10

WORKOUT
Run – 3 miles
Actual distance: 3.05 miles
Time: 20.52 minutes
Average pace: 6.57 m/m

Go straight from run into the weights training session.

WORKOUT
Weights (repeat cycle 4 times)
Squats: × 20
Static lunges: × 20
Frog jumps: × 20
Jumps overs: × 20
Calf raise: × 20

Squats bosu (upside down)
3 × 30 no weight

Squats with bar
3 × 30, 30kg

Squats bosu
3 × 30 no weight

Superset

	Glute extension	Dirty dogs
Sets and Reps	5 × 20	5 × 20

My notes: I ran as hard and as fast as I could, which made me feel sick at the end. The wind was against me on the way back, and when I was back in the gym I went straight into the weights. Loved today's session although it was really difficult. Stretched loads on my legs at the end of the session.

WORKOUT
Run – 3 miles
Actual distance: miles
Time: minutes
Average pace: m/m

WORKOUT
Weights (repeat cycle 4 times)
Squats: ×
Static lunges: ×
Frog jumps: ×
Jumps overs: ×
Calf raise: ×

Squats bosu (upside down)
×   no weight

Squats with bar
×   , 30kg

Squats bosu
×   no weight

Superset

	Glute extension	Dirty dogs
Sets and Reps	×	×

Your notes:

TRAINING SESSION **WEEK 9** DAY 5

MY TRAINING SESSION

AM Rest

PM **Training session** Weights – Chest and back; PT – Upper body

Time trained 6.15–7.20 p.m.

Session time 55 minutes

RPE 7/10

WORKOUT
WEIGHTS – CHEST AND BACK
Bench press
1 × 20 warm-up – with just Olympic bar
Set and Rep: 1. 20 2. 15 3. 10 4. 10 5. 10 6. 8 7. 6
Weight (lb): 40 50 70 90 100 110 115

Bent-over row
1 × 20 warm-up – with just Olympic bar
Set and Rep: 1. 20 2. 15 3. 10 4. 10 5. 10
Weight (lb): 30 50 90 90 90

PT – Upper body, chest and abs (repeat cycle 5 times)
Regular press-ups: × 15
½ sit-ups: × 15
Diamond press-ups: × 15
Leg levers: × 15
Wide push-ups: × 15
V sit-ups: × 15
Total press-ups: 225
Total sit-ups: 225

Arm haulers: × 45

My notes: no rest in between sets and reps on pull-ups, press-ups and sit-ups. Got a good pump on the press-ups after bench pressing 115kg.

YOUR TRAINING SESSION

AM

PM **Training session** Weights – Chest and back; PT – Upper body

Time trained

Session time

RPE /10

WORKOUT
WEIGHTS – CHEST AND BACK
Bench press
1 × 20 warm-up – with just Olympic bar
Set and Rep: 1. 2. 3. 4. 5. 6. 7.
Weight (kg):

Bent-over row
1 × 20 warm-up – with just Olympic bar
Set and Rep: 1. 2. 3. 4. 5.
Weight (kg):

PT – Upper body, chest and abs (repeat cycle 5 times)
Regular press-ups: ×
½ sit-ups: ×
Diamond press-ups: ×
Leg levers: ×
Wide push-ups: ×
V sit-ups: ×
Total press-ups:
Total sit-ups:

Arm haulers: ×

Your notes:

TRAINING SESSION **WEEK 9** DAY 6

MY TRAINING SESSION

AM Rest

PM Training session CV – Walk

Time trained 7.45–1.25 p.m.

Session time 4 hour 40 minutes

RPE 5/10

WORKOUT
Walk – 15 miles
Actual distance: 18.00 miles
Time: 4 hours 40 minutes
Average pace: 15.55 m/m

My equipment
Food:	2 bananas	2 apples
	1 bag soya nuts	1 bag goji berries
	3 turkey breasts	

My clothing:	Boots	Walking trousers
	Vest	Training top
	Walking socks	Waterproof jacket

Spare clothing:	Sandals	Warm jacket/top
	Gloves	Hat
	Scarf	

Other:	First-aid kit	Torch
	First field dressing	Map and compass
	Cycling shorts	Money
	Mobile phone	Whistle

My notes: you should all get out and walk more like this. I went with a friend for this walk. We had all the right equipment for any type of situation and weather. It was lucky for us that we did, because the heavens opened after an hour with torrential rain. Eventually the skies cleared and it turned out to be extremely sunny.

YOUR TRAINING SESSION

AM

PM Training session CV – Walk

Time trained

Session time

RPE /10

WORKOUT
Walk – 15 miles
Actual distance: miles
Time: minutes
Average pace: m/m

Your equipment
Food:

Your clothing:

Spare clothing:

Other:

Your notes:

WEEK 9 TESTS

Front view of me at the end of week 9.

Back view of me at the end of week 9.

MY WEEKLY TESTS

Weight (kg):   78.5
Height (cm):   175.5
BMI: 25.5
RHR: 40
BP: 135/46
Fat %:   13.2

Measurements (cm)
Neck: 38.10
Chest: 106.68
Arm: R 37.46   L 37.46
Navel: 78.74
Hips: 82.55
Thighs: R 61.59   L 61.59
Calves: R 40   L 40

YOUR WEEKLY TESTS

Weight (kg):
Height (cm):
BMI:
RHR:
BP:
Fat %:

Measurements (cm)
Neck:
Chest:
Arm: R   L
Navel:
Hips:
Thighs: R   L
Calves: R   L

WEEK TEN NUTRITION PLAN **WEEK 10**

WEEK 10 OVERVIEW

Day	Breakfast	Lunch	Dinner
1	Fruit porridge	Butternut squash and coriander soup	Swordfish with courgette salad
2	Fruit salad	Beetroot salad	Baked lamb and vegetables
3	Muesli with fresh fruit	Beef salad pitta	Poached chicken
4	Wheat biscuits or muesli with fruit	Chicken wrap	Marlin steaks
5	Fresh fruit and seeds	Tuna and olive salad	Baked Mediterranean vegetables with ricotta and turkey
6	Omelette	Vegetable soup	Monkfish delight
7	Fruit smoothie 1	Tuna salad	Garlic lamb

SHOPPING LIST WEEK 10

CARBOHYDRATES
1 bag of brown rice
1 bag of couscous
240g of muesli
560g porridge oats
1 bag of sunflower seeds
1 bag of pumpkin seeds
4 sweet potatoes
4 organic tortilla wraps
4 wholemeal/brown pitta
  breads
1 bag of wild rice
Wheat biscuits

DAIRY AND NON-DAIRY ALTERNATIVES
8 eggs
200g ricotta cheese/goat's
  cheese
680ml skimmed/soya/rice/
  oat milk
1.5kg soya yoghurt

FISH
8 anchovy fillets
350g cod or haddock
4 marlin steaks
350g monkfish
16 large raw prawns
4 × 200g swordfish steaks
350g tuna steaks
4 small tins of tuna

MEAT
400g cooked roast beef
8 chicken breasts
400g lean ham
350g boneless lamb
800g rack of lamb
4 turkey breasts

FRUIT
6 apples
1 apricot
8 bananas
1 punnet of blackberries
4 lemons
2 limes
2 mangos
2 oranges
1 peach
1 large pineapple
1 punnet of raspberries
1 watermelon

VEGETABLES
2 aubergines
200g baby carrots
4 cooked beetroots
1kg butternut squash
24 black olives
4 carrots
8 celery sticks
8 courgettes
1 cucumber
175g French beans
200g green beans
1 green pepper
2 lettuces
50g mangetout
6 onions
200g peas
4 red onions
4 red peppers
22 red tomatoes
115g baby plum tomatoes
100g rocket salad
4 shallots
10 spring onions
2 yellow peppers

HERBS
Basil
Black pepper
Chilli powder
Chives
Cinnamon sticks
Cumin
Fresh ginger
1 garlic bulb
1 green chilli
Mint
Nutmeg
Oregano
Paprika
Parsley
Rosemary
Tarragon
4 thyme sprigs
Turmeric

OTHER
150g dried apricots
Balsamic vinegar
Chicken stock
Chinese rice wine
Cold-pressed extra virgin
  olive oil
Dijon mustard
Fish stock
Honey
Light soy sauce
Plain flour
Soy sauce
Brown sugar
Tabasco sauce
400g tinned tomatoes
Vegetable stock

SNACKS
Fruit
Wholegrain crispbread
  crackers
Flat breads
Small bowl of muesli
Yoghurt/soya yoghurt
Nuts (cashew, pine or
  occasionally mixed nuts)
Soya nuts
Seeds (pumpkin or sunflower)

FRUIT DRINKS
1 carton fruit juice

RECIPES **WEEK 10** DAY 1

BREAKFAST FRUIT PORRIDGE   *See page 81*

LUNCH BUTTERNUT SQUASH
AND CORIANDER SOUP   *See page 88*

DINNER SWORDFISH WITH
COURGETTE SALAD

4 × 200g swordfish steaks

1 tablespoon olive oil

Lemon wedges

2 tablespoons fresh parsley, chopped

Couscous

For the salad:

2 teaspoons olive oil

2 tablespoons lemon juice

½ red onion, finely sliced

12 olives (optional)

3 small courgettes

1 To make salad, combine the olive oil, lemon juice, onion and olives in a bowl.
2 Steam the courgettes until tender.
3 Transfer to salad mixture and toss to coat.
4 Boil and cook couscous.
5 Heat a non-stick frying pan over a medium heat, brush swordfish steaks with oil and pan fry for 2 minutes on each side.
6 Toss the parsley through courgette salad and spoon on to serving plates.
7 Place swordfish on top of salad and serve with couscous, and lemon wedges to garnish.

RECIPES **WEEK 10** DAY 2

BREAKFAST FRUIT SALAD

See page 85

LUNCH BEETROOT SALAD

See page 97

DINNER BAKED LAMB AND VEGETABLES

1 tablespoon olive oil	**1** Preheat oven to 200°C (400°F).
4 thyme sprigs, chopped	**2** In a bowl mix half the oil with herbs, garlic and lemon zest.
1 tablespoon tarragon, chopped	**3** Heat a large frying pan over a high heat.
1 tablespoon parsley, chopped	**4** Coat lamb in remaining oil and sear until golden on both sides.
1 clove garlic	**5** Transfer to a baking dish, rub herb mixture into lamb rack and bake for 25 minutes.
800g rack of lamb (200g per person), fat removed	**6** Remove from oven, cover loosely with foil and set aside for 10 minutes.
1 lemon, zest finely grated	**7** Bring a large saucepan of water to the boil and cook carrots for 2 minutes, adding the beans and peas for a further 4 minutes.
200g baby carrots	**8** Drain and serve with the lamb.
200g green beans	
200g peas	

RECIPES **WEEK 10** DAY 3

BREAKFAST MUESLI WITH FRESH FRUIT

See page 80

LUNCH BEEF SALAD PITTA

See page 101

DINNER POACHED CHICKEN

2 tablespoons light soy sauce

1 tablespoon Chinese rice wine

2cm piece fresh ginger, sliced

1 tablespoon coriander

6 spring onions, finely sliced

1 litre of chicken stock

4 skinless chicken breasts

Brown rice and vegetables

1 In a large saucepan bring the soy sauce, Chinese rice wine, ginger, coriander, four of the spring onions and chicken stock to the boil.
2 Add the chicken, then reduce the heat and simmer for 12 minutes.
3 Remove from heat and allow chicken to rest in liquid for 5 minutes.
4 Slice chicken thickly and place on serving plate.
5 Pour liquid from saucepan over the chicken and sprinkle the rest of the spring onions over.
6 Serve with rice and vegetables.

Lunch for tomorrow:
CHICKEN WRAP
Consider preparing chicken in advance for tomorrow's lunch.

RECIPES **WEEK 10** DAY 4

BREAKFAST WHEAT BISCUITS OR MUESLI WITH FRUIT

See page 84

LUNCH CHICKEN WRAP

See page 113

DINNER MARLIN STEAKS

4 marlin steaks

For the dressing:

100ml olive oil

2 limes, juiced

1 clove of garlic, crushed

1 tablespoon parsley, of chopped

½ teaspoon dried oregano

1 tablespoon olive oil

Generous amounts of vegetables of your choice

1 For the dressing, place the olive oil in a mixing bowl and slowly whisk in 70ml of hot water and lime juice.
2 Add the garlic, parsley and oregano and whisk until smooth.
3 Heat the olive oil in a large frying pan on high heat.
4 Add the marlin steaks and cook for 3 minutes on each side.
5 Serve with vegetables and drizzle the dressing over the top.

RECIPES **WEEK 10** DAY 5

BREAKFAST FRESH FRUIT AND SEEDS

See page 82

LUNCH TUNA AND OLIVE SALAD

See page 81

DINNER BAKED MEDITERRANEAN VEGETABLES WITH RICOTTA AND TURKEY

1 red pepper, halved and deseeded

1 yellow pepper, halved and deseeded

4 courgettes, finely sliced lengthways

1 aubergine, finely sliced

1 tablespoon olive oil

1 clove garlic, crushed

2 small red onions, finely sliced

4 plum tomatoes, diced

115g fresh basil

200g low fat ricotta cheese or goat's cheese

4 turkey breasts

1 Preheat the oven to 180°C (350°F).
2 Place peppers, skin-side up, in a baking dish, drizzle with a little olive oil and roast for 20 minutes.
3 Remove from oven, cover with foil and allow to cool slightly.
4 Slice flesh into thick strips.
5 Preheat grill to high.
6 In a bowl toss the courgette and aubergine with half the oil. Grill vegetables until soft.
7 Heat the remaining oil in a large non-stick frying pan over a high heat. Add the garlic and onion and cook until soft.
8 Arrange vegetables, including tomatoes and basil, in layers in a non-stick baking dish.
9 Crumble ricotta cheese over the top and bake for 30 minutes.
10 Grill turkey breasts on medium heat for 8–12 minutes, or until cooked. Keep turning.
11 Serve the turkey with vegetables and ricotta cheese.

RECIPES **WEEK 10** DAY 6

BREAKFAST OMELETTE
See page 88

LUNCH VEGETABLE SOUP
See page 100

DINNER MONKFISH DELIGHT

16 large raw prawns, peeled

350g cod or haddock fillet, skinned and diced

350g monkfish, diced

2 onions, finely chopped

4 celery sticks, finely chopped

2 tablespoons plain flour

700ml fish stock

1 red pepper, deseeded and chopped

1 green pepper, deseeded and chopped

2 large tomatoes, chopped

1 tablespoon olive oil

1 garlic clove, crushed

½ teaspoon brown sugar

1 teaspoon ground cumin

4 tablespoons parsley, chopped

1 tablespoon fresh coriander, chopped

Dash Tabasco sauce

Brown or basmati rice

1. Heat the olive oil in a large saucepan. Add the onion and celery and cook for 5 minutes (stir occasionally).
2. Add the garlic and cook for 1 minute.
3. Next, stir in the flour, sugar and cumin and cook for 2 minutes – keep stirring.
4. Gradually stir in the fish stock and bring to the boil, stirring constantly.
5. Boil the rice.
6. Add the peppers and tomatoes to the saucepan and partially cover. Reduce the heat to very low and simmer gently for 10 minutes. Stir occasionally.
7. Add the parsley, coriander and Tabasco sauce and then gently stir in the fish and peeled prawns.
8. Cover and simmer gently for 5 minutes or until the fish is cooked through and the prawns have changed colour.
9. Gently mix and transfer to serving plates.
10. Serve with rice.

RECIPES **WEEK 10** DAY 7

BREAKFAST FRUIT SMOOTHIE 1   *See page 87*

LUNCH TUNA SALAD   *See page 131*

DINNER GARLIC LAMB

1 tablespoon olive oil

1 onion, chopped

350g lean boneless lamb, diced

600ml vegetable stock

1 orange, grated zest and juice

1 aubergine, halved lengthways and sliced thinly

4 tomatoes, chopped

115g no-soak dried apricots

1 garlic clove, finely chopped

1 teaspoon clear honey

1 cinnamon stick

1 cm piece ginger, finely chopped

2 tablespoons fresh coriander, chopped

Brown rice

1 Heat the olive oil in a large frying pan over a medium heat.
2 Add the onions and lamb cubes, stirring frequently, for 5 minutes, or until meat is slightly browned all over.
3 Add the garlic, vegetable stock, orange zest and juice, honey, cinnamon stick and ginger and bring to boil.
4 Reduce the heat, cover and simmer for 45 minutes.
5 Add the aubergine, tomatoes and apricots.
6 Cover and cook for a further 45 minutes, or until lamb is tender.
7 Stir in the coriander and season with black pepper.
8 Serve immediately with brown rice.

Lunch for tomorrow:
CHICKEN SALAD PITTA
Consider preparing chicken in advance.

TRAINING DIARY **WEEK 10**

WEEK 10 OVERVIEW
Day 1: Weights – Chest and back
Day 2: CV – Cycle; CV – Cycle; Weights – Shoulders and arms
Day 3: CV – Cycle; CV – Cycle; Cycle PT – Whole body
Day 4: Rest
Day 5: CV – Run; Weights – Chest and back
Day 6: CV – Run
Day 7: Rest
Any day: Myo stretch

MY DIARY
Day 1 (Monday)
It was a normal day today, and by the time I got into the gym and started with my pull-ups I noticed how easy it was and how much better I was at it. I can't wait for my final test day now, just to see how well I do.
Tiredness 3
Stress 2
Sleep 8 hours

Day 2 (Tuesday)
I'm going to do more cycling now, so I stayed over at Alison's and cycled to work from there as it's not as far as mine. I had a lymphatic massage today because I cycled home and I needed all the energy I could get.
Tiredness 3
Stress 3
Sleep 5 hours 30 minutes

Day 3 (Wednesday)
I cycled to work from my house in Hampshire to Poole. After my workout with a friend, I cycled back to Alison's house and finally had an evening doing nothing.
Tiredness 4
Stress 3
Sleep 5 hours 30 minutes

Day 4 (Thursday)
No training today, so I decided to make the most of this and had a massage. This was probably the best massage I've ever had, as it seemed to make me stand taller, my legs felt lighter and my back was much freer.
Tiredness 3
Stress 2
Sleep 7 hours

Day 5 (Friday)
As my body was feeling so good today my training was amazing. I lifted well and trained nice and hard.
Tiredness 3
Stress 2
Sleep 7 hours 30 minutes

Day 6 (Saturday)
I don't know why, but I had a choice between running 10 miles or kayaking over 5 hours from Barton on Sea to Poole Harbour along the coast – I chose the kayaking. It was a great experience.
Tiredness 2
Stress 0
Sleep 7 hours

Day 7 (Sunday)
I took the day off, and being the idiot I am I was sunburnt all over – very sore and tender. That will teach me to keep applying the sun cream while exercising outside. In the evening I had a BBQ at a friend's house.
Tiredness 3
Stress 1
Sleep 9 hours 15 minutes

TRAINING SESSION **WEEK 10** DAY 1

MY TRAINING SESSION

AM Rest

PM **Training session** Weights – Chest and back

Time trained 6.20–7.50 p.m.

Session time 1 hour 30 minutes

RPE 8/10

WORKOUT
Regular pull-ups
1–10 and 10–1
Total: 110

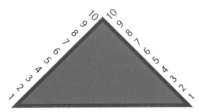

Incline fly
Set and Rep:	1. 15	2. 15	3. 10	4. 10	5. 9
Weight (lb):	35	45	55	55	55

Dumbbells bench press
Set and Rep:	1. 10	2. 10	3. 9	4. 9
Weight (lb):	50	60	70	70

Single arm row
Set and Rep:	1. 15	2. 10	3. 10	4. 10
Weight (lb):	70	80	90	90

Reverse shrug (dumb bell)
Set and Rep:	1. 20	2. 20	3. 20	4. 20
Weight (lb):	85	85	85	85

Morey squeeze (upper)
Set and Rep:	1. 10	2. 10	3. 10	4. 10
Weight (lb):	30	30	30	30

YOUR TRAINING SESSION

AM

PM **Training session** Weights – Chest and back

Time trained

Session time

RPE /10

WORKOUT
Regular pull-ups

Total:

Incline fly
Set and Rep:	1.	2.	3.	4.	5.
Weight (kg):					

Dumbbells bench press
Set and Rep:	1.	2.	3.	4.
Weight (kg):				

Single arm row
Set and Rep:	1.	2.	3.	4.
Weight (kg):				

Reverse shrug (dumb bell)
Set and Rep:	1.	2.	3.	4.
Weight (kg):				

Morey squeeze (upper)
Set and Rep:	1.	2.	3.	4.
Weight (kg):				

My notes: from 10 to 1 on the pull-ups, I put on an extra weight of 7.5kg to make my back work a lot harder.

Your notes:

TRAINING SESSION **WEEK 10** DAY 2

MY TRAINING SESSION

AM Rest

PM Training session CV – Cycle

Time trained 5.11–6.13 p.m.

Session time 1 hour 2 minutes

RPE 9/10

PM Training session Weights – Shoulders and arms

Time trained 6.25–7.25 p.m.

Session time 1 hour

RPE 8/10

WORKOUT
Cycle – 20 miles
Actual distance: 19.70 miles

YOUR TRAINING SESSION

AM

PM Training session CV – Cycle

Time trained

Session time

RPE /10

PM Training session Weights – Shoulders and arms

Time trained

Session time

RPE /10

WORKOUT
Cycle – 20 miles
Actual distance: miles

Go straight into the weights as quick as you can.

Dumbbell press

1 × 20 warm-up

Set and Rep:	1. 20	2. 10	3. 10	4. 6	5. 7
Weight (lb):	35	45	55	55	55

Front arm raise (alternate)

Set and Rep:	1. 10	2. 8	3. 10
Weight (lb):	25	25	25

Triceps press-downs (reverse grip)

Set and Rep:	1. 10	2. 8	3. 8	4. 8
Weight (kg):	25	25	25	25

Supernated curl – drop bench

90, 75, 60, 45

Set and Rep:	1. 10	2. 10	3. 6	4. 6
Weight (lb):	35	35	35	35

Superset

	Lat raise			Bent-over lat raise		
Set and Rep:	1. 10	2. 10	3. 10	1. 10	2. 10	3. 10
Weight (kg)	25	25	25	25	25	25

Superset

	Preacher curl			Single arm pull-down		
Set and Rep:	1. 10	2. 10	3. 10	1. 15	2. 15	3. 15
Weight (kg)	35	35	35	7.5	7.5	7.5

My notes: all I can say is good luck for training today. It was hard work, but it's an amazing feeling when you finish.

Dumbbell press

1 × 20 warm-up

Set and Rep:	1.	2.	3.	4.	5.
Weight (kg):					

Front arm raise (alternate)

Set and Rep:	1.	2.	3.
Weight (kg):			

Triceps press-downs (reverse grip)

Set and Rep:	1.	2.	3.	4.
Weight (kg):				

Supernated curl – drop bench

, , ,

Set and Rep:	1.	2.	3.	4.
Weight (kg):				

Superset

	Lat raise			Bent-over lat raise		
Set and Rep:	1.	2.	3.	1.	2.	3.
Weight (kg):						

Superset

	Preacher curl			Single arm pull-down		
Set and Rep:	1.	2.	3.	1.	2.	3.
Weight (kg):						

Your notes:

TRAINING SESSION **WEEK 10** DAY 3

MY TRAINING SESSION

AM Training session CV – Cycle

Time trained 7.40–8.43 a.m.

Session time 1 hour 03 minutes

RPE 8/10

PM Training session Cycle PT – Whole body

Time trained 7.00–7.50 p.m.

Session time 50 minutes

RPE 7/10

WORKOUT
Cycle – 20 miles
Actual Distance: 19.70 miles

Cycle PT
Cycle distance: 7 miles

Cycle 3 miles to Station 1

Station 1 (repeat cycle 10 times)
Dips: × 10
½ sit-ups: × 20
Press-ups: × 10
Pull-ups: × 10

Cycle 3 miles to Station 2

YOUR TRAINING SESSION

AM Training session CV – Cycle

Time trained

Session time

RPE /10

PM Training session Cycle PT – Whole body

Time trained

Session time

RPE /10

WORKOUT
Cycle – 20 miles
Actual distance: miles

Cycle PT
Cycle distance: miles

Cycle 3 miles to Station 1

Station 1 (repeat cycle 10 times)
Dips: ×
½ sit-ups: ×
Press-ups: ×
Pull-ups: ×

Cycle 3 miles to Station 2

Station 2 (repeat cycle 5 times)
Dips: × 10
½ sit-ups: × 10
Press-ups wide: × 10
Pull-ups: × 10

Cycle 1 mile to finish

My notes: from 10 to 1 on the pull-ups, I put on an extra weight of 7.5kg to make my back work a lot harder.

Station 2 (repeat cycle 5 times)
Dips: ×
½ sit-ups: ×
Press-ups wide: ×
Pull-ups: ×

Cycle 1 mile to finish

Your notes:

TRAINING SESSION **WEEK 10** DAY 5

MY TRAINING SESSION

AM **Training session** CV – Run

Time trained 11.00–11.30 a.m.

Session time 30 minutes

RPE 6/10

PM **Training session** Weights – Chest and back

Time trained 6.20–8.00 p.m.

Session time 1 hour 40 minutes

RPE 7/10

YOUR TRAINING SESSION

AM **Training session** CV – Run

Time trained

Session time

RPE   /10

PM **Training session** Weights – Chest and back

Time trained

Session time

RPE   /10

WORKOUT
Run – 3 miles
Actual distance: 3.05 miles
Time: 24 minutes
Average Pace: 8.00 m/m

Incline bench press
1 × 20 warm-up – with just Olympic bar

Set and Rep:	1. 10	2. 10	3. 10	4. 8	5. 7
Weight (kg):	50	70	90	100	100

Decline bench press

Set and Rep:	1. 10	2. 10	3. 6	4. 6
Weight (kg):	100	110	120	120

T-bar row

Set and Rep:	1. 10	2. 10	3. 10	4. 10
Weight (kg):	55	75	90	90

Deadlifts
1 × 20 warm-up – with just Olympic bar

Set and Rep:	1. 10	2. 10	3. 10	4. 8
Weight (kg):	70	110	120	120

Pec fly

Set and Rep:	1. 10	2. 10	3. 10
Weight (lb):	65	65	65

My notes: this was the one workout where I felt the strongest. It was a hard and long session, but I pushed as much weight as possible while keeping perfect form.

WORKOUT
Run – 3 miles
Actual distance: miles
Time: minutes
Average Pace: m/m

Incline bench press
1 × 20 warm-up – with just Olympic bar

Set and Rep:	1.	2.	3.	4.	5.
Weight (kg):					

Decline bench press

Set and Rep:	1.	2.	3.	4.
Weight (kg):				

T-bar row

Set and Rep:	1.	2.	3.	4.
Weight (kg):				

Deadlifts
1 × 20 warm-up – with just Olympic bar

Set and Rep:	1.	2.	3.	4.
Weight (kg):				

Pec fly

Set and Rep:	1.	2.	3.
Weight (kg):			

Your notes:

TRAINING SESSION **WEEK 10** DAY 6

MY TRAINING SESSION

AM/PM Training session CV – Run (or Kayak)

Time trained 11.15–4.30 p.m.

Session time 5 hours 40 minutes

RPE 10/10

WORKOUT
Kayak – 15 miles
Actual distance: 18.25 miles
Time: 5 hours 15 minutes
Average pace: 17.26 m/m

My equipment
Food:	2 oranges	2 apples
	1 bag soy nuts	2 corn on cob
	3 mackerel	3 litres of water
My clothing:	Buffalo warm jacket	Gloves
	Cycling shorts	Hat
	Scarf	Training top
	Wet suit	Life jacket
In my dry bag:	Sandals	First-aid kit
	Torch	Map
	Compass	Money
	Mobile phone	Trolley
	iPod and speakers	Whistle

My notes: this is what outdoor training is all about. The weather and sea conditions couldn't have been better. I ran a one mile round trip to see what the sea conditions were like, then packed up all my stuff and walked about one mile pulling my kayak along with its trolley. I only got caught twice with the current, one at Hengsbury Head and the other in Poole Harbour, which was really strong. I got sunburnt, although I'd put on factor 15 lotion. There wasn't much I could do about it because I'd forgotten to take the sun cream with me.

YOUR TRAINING SESSION

AM/PM Training session CV – Run (or Kayak)

Time trained

Session time

RPE /10

WORKOUT
Run – 10 miles (or kayak – 15 miles)
Actual distance: miles
Time: minutes
Average pace: m/m

Your equipment
Food:

Spare clothing:

Other:

Your notes:

WEEK 10 TESTS

Front view of me at the end of week 10.

Back view of me at the end of week 10.

MY WEEKLY TESTS

Weight (kg):   78.5
Height (cm): 175.5
BMI: 25.5
RHR: 40
BP: 140/45
Fat %:   13.1

Measurements (cm)
Neck: 38.10
Chest: 106.68
Arm: R 37.46   L 37.46
Navel: 78.74
Hips: 81.91
Thighs: R 61.59   L 61.59
Calves: R 40   L 40

YOUR WEEKLY TESTS

Weight (kg):
Height (cm):
BMI:
RHR:
BP:
Fat %:

Measurements (cm)
Neck:
Chest:
Arm: R   L
Navel:
Hips:
Thighs: R   L
Calves: R   L

WEEK **ELEVEN** NUTRITION PLAN **WEEK 11**

WEEK 11 OVERVIEW

Day	Breakfast	Lunch	Dinner
1	Fresh fruit and seeds	Chicken salad pitta	Fennel and halibut parcels
2	Scrambled eggs with wild mushrooms	Tuna salad	Mint chicken and lime
3	Muesli and fresh fruit	Yellow split pea soup	Mango and rum snapper
4	Fruit porridge	Salmon salad	Stuffed peppers
5	Fruit salad	Egg salad	Lamb curry with spinach
6	Omelette	Tomato and pepper soup	Hungarian goulash
7	Fruit smoothie 1	Chicken wrap	Chilli prawn salad

SHOPPING LIST **WEEK 11**

CARBOHYDRATES
1 bag of couscous
240g of muesli
560g porridge oats
1 bag of sunflower seeds
1 bag of pumpkin seeds
225g yellow split peas
5 sweet potatoes
4 organic tortilla wraps
4 wholemeal/brown pitta
  breads
1 bag of wild rice
Wheat biscuits

DAIRY AND NON-DAIRY ALTERNATIVES
13 eggs
40g feta/goats cheese
280g low fat fromage frais
680ml skimmed/soya/rice/
  oat milk
2kg soya yoghurt

FISH
8 anchovy fillets
4 halibut steaks
200g jumbo raw prawns
4 poached salmon fillets
500g red snapper
4 tins of tuna

MEAT
8 chicken breasts
8 boneless chicken thighs
800g lean braising streaks
400g lean ham
800g lean lamb leg

FRUIT
6 apples
2 apricot
10 bananas
1 punnet of blackberries
4 lemons
2 limes
3 mangos
1 melon
2 oranges
3 peaches
1 punnet of raspberries

VEGETABLES
1 avocado
1 baby gem lettuce
600g baby spinach
125g broccoli
12 button mushrooms
3 carrots
8 celery sticks
400g cherry tomatoes
2 cos lettuce
3 courgettes
1 cucumber
1 fennel bulb
2 green peppers
2 leeks
2 lettuces
50g mangetout
8 large wild mushrooms
335g mushrooms
8 onions
1 red onion
5 red peppers
18 red tomatoes
100g rocket salad
10 spring onions
750g tomatoes
10 yellow peppers

HERBS
Basil
1 bay leaf
Black pepper
Caraway seeds
Cardamon seeds
Chives
Ground cinnamon
Cumin
Garam masala
Fresh ginger
1 garlic bulb
Marjoram
Mint
Paprika
Parsley
2 red chillies
Thyme
Turmeric

OTHER
Balsamic vinegar
Cider vinegar
Cold-pressed extra virgin
  olive oil
Dijon mustard
Fish stock
Honey
Plain flour
Dark rum
800g tinned tomatoes
Tomato purée
Vegetable stock
75ml white wine

SNACKS
Fruit
Wholegrain crispbread
  crackers
Flat breads
Small bowl of muesli
Yoghurt/soya yoghurt
Nuts (cashew, pine or
  occasionally mixed nuts)
Soya nuts
Seeds (pumpkin or sunflower)

FRUIT DRINKS
1 carton fruit juice

RECIPES **WEEK 11** DAY 1

BREAKFAST FRESH FRUIT AND SEEDS

See page 82

LUNCH CHICKEN SALAD PITTA

See page 120

DINNER FENNEL AND HALIBUT PARCELS

4 halibut steaks (175g each)

2 leeks, cut into thin strips

2 courgettes, cut into thin slices

2 carrots, cut into thin slices

1 fennel bulb, halved and cut into thin strips

115g/4oz mushrooms, thinly sliced

4 teaspoons olive oil

4 tablespoons white wine

Vegetables of your choice

1 Preheat oven to 190°C (375°F).
2 Cut out four 30cm squares of baking paper and spread out on a work surface.
3 Divide the leeks, courgettes, carrots, fennel and mushroom equally between the paper squares.
4 Top each bed of vegetables with a halibut steak.
5 Fold up the edges of the paper, but do not seal.
6 Drizzle 1 teaspoon of olive oil and 1 tablespoon of white wine over each fish steak.
7 Fold over the edges of the paper to seal to make a loosely wrapped parcel.
8 Place the parcels on a large baking sheet and bake in the oven for 10–15 minutes or until parcels are puffed and fish is cooked.
9 Transfer to plates and serve with vegetables.

Lunch for tomorrow:
TUNA SALAD
Consider preparing sweet potatoes your lunch in advance.

RECIPES **WEEK 11** DAY 2

BREAKFAST SCRAMBLED EGGS
WITH WILD MUSHROOMS

See page 99

LUNCH TUNA SALAD

See page 131

DINNER MINT CHICKEN AND LIME

8 lean, boneless chicken thighs

Salad of your choice

For the marinade:

3 tablespoons fresh mint, finely chopped

4 tablespoons clear honey

2 tablespoons lime juice

For the sauce:

150g low fat natural soya/plain yoghurt

1 tablespoon fresh mint, finely chopped

2 teaspoons lime zest, finely grated

1 Mix the honey, mint and lime juice in a large bowl.
2 Add chicken to marinade and evenly coat both sides.
3 Cover with cling film and leave the chicken to refrigerate for at least 30 minutes, longer if possible.
4 Remove the chicken and reserve the marinade. Preheat the grill to medium.
5 Place the chicken on the grill tray and cook under a hot grill for 15–18 minutes, or until chicken is tender and cooked. Turn the chicken frequently and keep covering chicken with marinade.
6 Meanwhile, mix all the sauce ingredients together in a bowl.
7 Serve the chicken with the salad and use the remaining marinade for dipping.

Lunch for tomorrow:
YELLOW SPLIT PEA SOUP
Pre-soak the yellow split peas overnight in cold water.

RECIPES **WEEK 11** DAY 3

BREAKFAST MUESLI WITH
FRESH FRUIT

See page 80

LUNCH YELLOW SPLIT PEA SOUP

See page 146

DINNER MANGO AND
RUM SNAPPER

2 tablespoons dark rum

50ml white wine

1 tablespoon ginger, finely chopped

1 clove garlic, finely chopped

500g red snapper fillets, cut into 4cm pieces

1 onion, cut into wedges

1 tablespoon olive oil

2 tablespoons plain flour

2 teaspoons tomato purée

500ml fish stock

2 large tomatoes, roughly chopped

1 mango, peeled, stoned
and roughly chopped

1 red pepper, deseeded and roughly chopped

Basmati rice

1 Mix the rum, wine, ginger and garlic in a large, shallow, non-metallic dish and add the fish to the marinade.
2 Cover with cling film and leave in the refrigerator to marinate for 30 minutes. Remove using a slotted spoon and reserve the marinade.
3 Boil the rice.
4 Heat the olive oil in a large saucepan, add the onion wedges and cook over a medium heat, stirring occasionally for 5 minutes.
5 Stir in the flour and add the tomato purée and red pepper.
6 Gradually stir in the fish stock and the reserved marinade and bring to boil, stirring continuously.
7 Reduce the heat and simmer for a further 3 minutes.
8 Add the fish, tomatoes and mango to the saucepan and cover.
9 Simmer for 8 minutes or until fish is cooked, then serve with rice.

RECIPES **WEEK 11** DAY 4

BREAKFAST FRUIT PORRIDGE   *See page 81*

LUNCH SALMON SALAD   *See page 118*

DINNER STUFFED PEPPERS

4 yellow peppers, halved lengthways and deseeded

150g baby spinach leaves

1 tablespoon olive oil

1 small onion, finely chopped

2 cloves garlic, crushed

3 tomatoes, chopped

12 button mushrooms, sliced

1 egg, lightly beaten

40g feta/goat's or mature cheese

2 tablespoons basil

Brown rice

1 Preheat oven to 180°C (350°F).
2 Heat the olive oil in a medium frying pan over a high heat and add the onions, garlic, tomatoes, mushrooms and spinach leaves and cook for 5 minutes, or until vegetables are soft.
3 Transfer to a large bowl and allow to cool slightly.
4 Add the egg and 1 tablespoon of water, and stir to combine.
5 Spoon the mixture into peppers and sprinkle the tops with cheese and basil.
6 Place peppers on baking tray and bake for 15–20 minutes, or until peppers are soft and cheese is slightly brown. Serve immediately with rice.

Lunch for tomorrow:
EGG SALAD
Consider preparing the eggs in advance.

RECIPES **WEEK 11 DAY 5**

BREAKFAST FRUIT SALAD

See page 85

LUNCH EGG SALAD

See page 116

DINNER LAMB CURRY WITH SPINACH

800g lean lamb leg, diced

2 tablespoons olive oil

2 onions, finely sliced

2 cloves garlic

115g soya/plain yoghurt

1 tin of chopped tomatoes

250g spinach

Fresh coriander, handful

Brown rice

Spices:

½ teaspoon cardamom seeds

1 teaspoon ground cinnamon

1 tablespoon garam masala

2 teaspoon turmeric

1 Heat olive oil in a large saucepan over a high heat and add the onion and garlic.
2 Cook for 5 minutes, or until onion is golden.
3 Add the spices and lamb, mix well and cook for 6–8 minutes, or until lamb begins to cook and change colour.
4 Stir through yoghurt and tomato.
5 Add spinach and 225ml of water, then reduce heat to medium and simmer for 40 minutes, or until meat is tender.
6 Stir through the coriander.
7 Serve with rice.

RECIPES **WEEK 11** DAY 6

BREAKFAST OMELETTE   *See page 88*

LUNCH TOMATO AND PEPPER SOUP   *See page 135*

DINNER HUNGARIAN GOULASH

800g lean braising steak

400g tinned chopped tomatoes

2 onions, finely chopped

220g mushrooms, sliced

2 green peppers, deseeded and diced

280g low fat fromage frais

Florets of broccoli

125g of peas

Brown rice

Herbs:

1 bay leaf

Marjoram, pinch

Thyme, pinch

2 level tablespoons paprika

¼ level teaspoon caraway seeds

1 Preheat oven to 150°C (300°F).
2 Place onions and tomatoes in pan and cook until onions are soft.
3 Add the mushrooms and peppers and cook for a further 5 minutes.
4 Cut the steak into strips and place in a casserole dish, adding the herbs and tomato mixture.
5 Cover and cook for about 1 hour 30 minutes.
6 Beat the fromage frais until smooth and pour over the casserole dish before serving.
7 Serve with the vegetables and brown rice.

RECIPES **WEEK 11** DAY 7

BREAKFAST FRUIT SMOOTHIE 1   *See page 87*

LUNCH CHICKEN WRAP   *See page 113*

DINNER CHILLI PRAWN SALAD

200g jumbo raw prawns

Handful fresh coriander

4 teaspoons lemon juice

1 yellow pepper

1 tablespoon olive oil

1cm ginger, peeled and finely chopped

2 cloves garlic, finely chopped

For the salad:

2 cos lettuces, torn into pieces

3–4 spring onions, finely sliced

2 fresh red chillies, deseeded and finely sliced

4 large tomatoes, sliced

1 Place the lettuce in a salad bowl, add the spring onions, tomatoes and yellow pepper and toss together.
2 Heat half of the olive oil in a large frying pan on a high heat.
3 Add the ginger, garlic, chillies and prawns.
4 Cook for 3 minutes, then reduce heat and squeeze the juice of a lemon over the frying pan.
5 Add the coriander, the rest of the olive oil and cook for a further minute.
6 Remove from the heat and season with black pepper.
7 Pour the prawn mixture over the salad and serve.

**Lunch for tomorrow:
TUNA SALAD**
Consider preparing the sweet potatoes in advance (refrigerate overnight).

TRAINING DIARY **WEEK 11**

WEEK 11 OVERVIEW
Day 1: CV – Cycle PT
Day 2: Weights – Chest and back
Day 3: CV – Run; CV – Cycle; PT – Legs
Day 4: CV – Cycle; CV – Cycle; PT – Upper body
Day 5: CV – Walk
Day 6: CV – Walk
Day 7: Weights – Whole body
Any day: Myo stretch

MY DIARY

Day 1 (Monday)
I did an amazing Cycle PT today, which pushed my training partner and me hard. I love these training sessions with other people as you get more out of the training, in various ways.
Tiredness 3
Stress 2
Sleep 8 hours

Day 2 (Tuesday)
I can't have a massage at the moment as I'm still a little sunburnt, but as soon as that goes I'm going to get a myo massage. I tried to work out for lunch but ran out of time, and when I got back from work I only had one hour to get out and have dinner at a client's house. I managed a 45-minute workout and still got there in time.
Tiredness 4
Stress 3
Sleep 6 hours 45 minutes

Day 3 (Wednesday)
I'm now peeling slightly on my shoulders so I chose to have a massage. This should shift all my dead skin as well as get me into shape for next week's tests.
Tiredness 4
Stress 3
Sleep 7 hours 30 minutes

Day 4 (Thursday)
I'm really enjoying the intensity of the training now, I can see such an improvement. I had a bright idea to take Alison away on a last-minute holiday to the south of France for her birthday, and I only had tonight to book it as we are going off tomorrow.
Tiredness 3
Stress 3
Sleep 7 hours

Day 5 (Friday)
I eventually got to bed at about 1.30 a.m. and surprised Alison at 5.00 a.m. in the morning to tell her we were off on holiday. She didn't know where she was going until we had to check in, which was a great surprise for her.
Tiredness 3
Stress 3
Sleep 3 hours

Day 6 (Saturday)
Walked around Nice, Antibes etc. and did some of the touristy things. It's a lovely place.
Tiredness 0
Stress 0
Sleep 7 hours

Day 7 (Sunday)
I got up early in the morning to use the hotel's gym before taking in more of the sights. I'm so happy to be on holiday, as this is the first time I have been away in over two years.
Tiredness 2
Stress 0
Sleep 7 hours

TRAINING SESSION **WEEK 11** DAY 1

MY TRAINING SESSION

AM Rest

PM Training session CV – Cycle PT

Time trained 5.40–6.55 p.m.

Session time 1 hour 15 minutes

RPE 9/10

WORKOUT

Perform the cycle first for 2 minutes 30 seconds with the level specified to make the cycle hard or easy (as the session continues the cycle resistance level also increases). Move on to the exercises. Complete all three sets and reps specified. No rest at all between any exercises or cycles. Average RPM: 100–120

Cycle – level 1 (easy)

Dumbbell press
Set and Rep:	1. 30	2. 20	3. 10
Weight (lb):	15	30	55

Cycle – level 2

Bent-over row
Set and Rep:	1. 30	2. 20	3. 10
Weight (lb):	20	45	70

Cycle – level 3

Incline fly
Set and Rep:	1. 30	2. 20	3. 10
Weight (lb):	20	35	55

Cycle – level 4

V sit-ups
Set and Rep:	1. 30	2. 20	3. 10

YOUR TRAINING SESSION

AM

PM Training session CV – Cycle PT

Time trained

Session time

RPE /10

WORKOUT

You should aim for 30 reps for the 1st set (easy weight), then 20 reps for the 2nd set (moderate weight) and finally 10 reps for the 3rd set (heavy weight).

Cycle – level 1 (easy)

Dumbbell press
Set and Rep:	1.	2.	3.
Weight (kg):			

Cycle – level 2

Bent-over row
Set and Rep:	1.	2.	3.
Weight (kg):			

Cycle – level 3

Incline fly
Set and Rep:	1.	2.	3.
Weight (kg):			

Cycle – level 4

V sit-ups
Set and Rep:	1.	2.	3.

Cycle – level 5

Bent-over lat raise

Set and Rep:	1. 30	2. 20	3. 10
Weight (lb):	15	25	35

Cycle – level 6

Regular press-ups

Set and Rep:	1. 30	2. 20	3. 10

Cycle – level 7

Reverse curls

Set and Rep:	1. 30	2. 20	3. 10

Cycle – level 8

Supernated curl

Set and Rep:	1. 30	2. 20	3. 10
Weight (lb):	15	25	35

Cycle – level 9

Dips

Set and Rep:	1. 30	2. 20	3. 10

Cycle – level 10
RPM: 60

Plank

Set and Rep:	1. 30	2. 20	3. 10

Rest for 2 – 5 minutes, then:

Pull-ups: 3 × 10

My notes: a brilliant all over workout that is fast and hard. I tried to use the heaviest weights for the 2nd and 3rd sets. I felt my sun burn a little bit on my shoulders though.

Cycle – level 5

Bent-over lat raise

Set and Rep: 1.	2.	3.
Weight (kg):		

Cycle – level 6

Regular press-ups

Set and Rep: 1.	2.	3.

Cycle – level 7

Reverse curls

Set and Rep: 1.	2.	3.

Cycle – level 8

Supernated curl

Set and Rep: 1.	2.	3.
Weight (kg):		

Cycle – level 9

Dips

Set and Rep: 1.	2.	3.

Cycle – level 10
RPM:

Plank

Set and Rep: 1.	2.	3.

Rest for 2 – 5 minutes, then:

Pull-ups: ×

Your notes:

TRAINING SESSION **WEEK 11** DAY 2

MY TRAINING SESSION

AM Rest

PM Training session Weights – Chest and back

Time trained 5.45–6.30 p.m.

Session time 45 minutes

RPE 9/10

WORKOUT

Superset	*Bench press*				*Incline dumbbell press*			
Sets	1.	2.	3.	4.	1.	2.	3.	4
Reps	10	10	9	9	10	10	9	9
Weight (kg)	35	40	40	40	55	65	65	65

Perform the supersets by completing all five pull-ups with two reps for each type, and once you have finished move on to the single arm row. Complete the first set, then go back and do all five pull-up types for the 2nd set followed by the 2nd set of single arm rows.

Superset

	Pull-ups	*Single arm row (40kg)*
Sets	Regular 4 × 2 reps	1. 10
and	Reverse 4 × 2 reps	2. 10
Reps	Close 4 × 2 reps	3. 10
	Wide 4 × 2 reps	4. 10
	Mountain climbers 4 × 2 reps	

My notes: this was quite hard and fast again, because I had time restraints. I superseded everything with almost no rest between the sets so I could do more exercise.

YOUR TRAINING SESSION

AM

PM Training session Weights – Chest and back

Time trained

Session time

RPE   /10

WORKOUT

Superset	*Bench press*				*Incline dumbbell press*			
Sets	1.	2.	3.	4.	1.	2.	3.	4.
Reps								
Weight (kg)								

Superset

	Pull-ups	*Single arm row (40kg)*
Sets	Regular	× 2 reps	1.
and	Reverse	× 2 reps	2.
Reps	Close	× 2 reps	3.
	Wide	× 2 reps	4.
	Mountain climbers × 2 reps	

Your notes:

TRAINING SESSION **WEEK 11** DAY 3

MY TRAINING SESSION

AM Training session CV – Run

Time trained 7.20–8.24 a.m.

Session time 1 hour 04 minutes

RPE 10/10

PM Training session CV – Cycle

Time trained 5.15–6.20 p.m.

Session time 1 hour 05 minutes

RPE 10/10

PM Training session PT – Legs

Time trained 7.20–8.24 a.m.

Session time 1 hour 04 minutes

RPE 10/10

YOUR TRAINING SESSION

AM Training session CV – Run

Time trained

Session time

RPE /10

PM Training session CV – Cycle

Time trained

Session time

RPE /10

PM Training session PT – Legs

Time trained

Session time

RPE /10

WORKOUT
Run – 8 miles
Actual distance: 8 Miles
Average pace: 8 m / m

Cycle – 20 miles
Actual distance: 19.70 miles

PT – Legs
Squats: 2 × 30
Single side squats on box: 3 × 30 (18kg)
Lunges on box: 3 × 30

WORKOUT
Run – 8 miles
Actual distance: miles
Average pace: m/m

Cycle – 20 miles
Actual distance: miles

PT – Legs
Squats: ×
Single side squats on box: ×   (kg)
Lunges on box: ×

Standing glute extensions: 3 × 30
Standing dirty dogs: 3 × 30
Squats: 3 × 30

Pull-ups
Regular pull-ups: 3 – 2 – 1
Reverse pull-ups: 3 – 2 – 1
Close pull-ups: 3 – 2 – 1
Wide pull-ups: 3 – 2 – 1
Mountain climber pull-ups: 3 – 2 – 1

My notes: the wind and rain was extreme today – it was in my face all of the way on the run, which didn't hold up once. I pushed it really hard so I didn't lose too much time.

The cycle home took much longer, which was no surprise because the wind was still against me. By the end I had nothing to give, so when I got back I ate some food and had a lot of water.

I did all of the pull-ups without putting my feet on floor to change hand positions, which made them much more difficult.

Standing glute extensions: ×
Standing dirty dogs: ×
Squats: ×

Pull-ups
Regular pull-ups: –   –
Reverse pull-ups: –   –
Close pull-ups: –   –
Wide pull-ups: –   –
Mountain climber pull-ups: –   –

Your notes:

TRAINING SESSION **WEEK 11** DAY 4

MY TRAINING SESSION

AM **Training session** CV – Cycle

Time trained 8.00–8.22 a.m.

Session time 22 minutes

RPE 10/10

YOUR TRAINING SESSION

AM **Training session** CV – Cycle

Time trained

Session time

RPE   /10

PM Training session CV – Cycle

Time trained 4.00–4.20 p.m.

Session time 20 minutes

RPE 10/10

PM Training session CV – Cycle

Time trained

Session time

RPE /10

PM Training session PT – Upper body

Time trained 4.20–4.55 p.m.

Session time 35 minutes

RPE 10/10

PM Training session PT – Upper body

Time trained

Session time

RPE /10

WORKOUT

Cycle – 10 miles
Actual distance: 8.2 Miles

Cycle – 10 miles
Actual distance: 8.2 miles

PT – Upper body
Chest and abs cycle (repeat 15 times)
Regular press-ups: × 15
½ sit-ups: × 15
Diamond press-ups: × 15
Leg levers: × 15
Wide push-ups: × 15
Reverse crunch: × 15
Total press-ups: 675
Total sit-ups: 675

My notes: finally the weather has been good to me for cycling. My legs seemed to fail quite quickly on the cycle home, which made the cycle a bit tougher. The PT upper body was relatively easy considering I went straight into it after the cycle.

WORKOUT

Cycle – 10 miles
Actual distance: miles

Cycle – 10 miles
Actual distance: miles

PT – Upper body
Chest and abs cycle (repeat 15 times)
Regular press-ups: ×
½ sit-ups: ×
Diamond press-ups: ×
Leg levers: ×
Wide push-ups: ×
Reverse crunch: ×
Total press-ups:
Total sit-ups:

Your notes:

TRAINING SESSION **WEEK 11** DAY 5

MY TRAINING SESSION

AM Rest

PM **Training session** CV – Walk

Time trained 1.00–4.05 p.m.

Session time 3 hour

RPE 4/10

WORKOUT
Walk – 10 miles
Actual distance: 8 miles
Time: 3 hours

My equipment
Food: 2 bananas
           2 apples
           2 oranges
Other: Mobile phone
           First-aid kit
           Money
Clothes: Shorts
           T-Shirt
           Socks
           Trainers

My notes: this walk was in the south of France in Nice. I find that the best way to see a place is to walk everywhere, so that is what we did. The weather was amazing. This walk was fairly easy, with a lunch in the middle and obviously some sightseeing. It was a fantastic break away, just what I needed.

YOUR TRAINING SESSION

AM

PM **Training session** CV – Walk

Time trained

Session time

RPE   /10

WORKOUT
Walk – 10 miles
Actual distance: miles
Time: hours

Your equipment
Food:

Other:

Clothes:

Your notes:

TRAINING SESSION **WEEK 11** DAY 6

MY TRAINING SESSION

AM Rest

PM Training session CV – Walk

Time trained all day

Session time 2 hour 30 minutes

RPE 4/10

WORKOUT
Walk – 10 miles
Actual distance: 6 miles
Time: 2 hours 30 minutes

My equipment
Food: 2 bananas
          2 apples
          2 bottles of water
Other: Mobile phone
          First-aid kit
          Money
Clothes: Shorts
          T-Shirt
          Sandals

My notes: another fantastic day for the weather. Again, we did lots of sightseeing.

YOUR TRAINING SESSION

AM

PM Training session CV – Walk

Time trained

Session time

RPE /10

WORKOUT
Walk – 10 miles
Actual distance: miles
Time: hours   minutes

Your equipment
Food:

Other:

Clothes:

Your notes:

TRAINING SESSION **WEEK 11** DAY 7

MY TRAINING SESSION

AM Training session Weights – Whole body

Time trained 7.30–8.30 p.m.

Session time 1 hour

RPE 8/10

PM Rest

WORKOUT
Warm-up on both exercises in the supersets with 20 reps before beginning.

Superset

	Bench press				Bent-over row			
Sets	1.	2.	3.	4.	1.	2.	3.	4
Reps	10	10	10	10	10	10	10	10
Weight (kg)	70	90	110	110	40	60	80	90

Superset

	Incline fly			Lat pull-down (close grip)		
Set and Rep	1. 10	2. 10	3. 10	1. 10	2. 10	3. 10
Weight (kg)	25	25	25	60	60	60

Superset

	Lat raise (cable)			Front arm raise (cable)		
Set and Rep	1. 10	2. 10	3. 10	1. 10	2. 10	3. 10
Weight (kg)	15	15	15	12.5	12.5	12.5

Superset

	Single-arm pull-downs			Supernated curl		
Sets and Rep	1. 10	2. 10	3. 10	1. 10	2. 10	3. 10
Weight (kg)	15	15	15	25	25	25

YOUR TRAINING SESSION

PM Training session Weights – Whole body

Time trained

Session time

RPE /10

PM

WORKOUT

Superset

	Bench press				Bent-over row			
Sets	1.	2.	3.	4.	1.	2.	3.	4.
Reps								
Weight (kg)								

Superset

	Incline fly			Lat pull-down (close grip)		
Set and Rep:	1.	2.	3.	1.	2.	3.
Weight (kg):						

Superset

	Lat raise (cable)			Front arm raise (cable)		
Set and Rep:	1.	2.	3.	1.	2.	3.
Weight (kg):						

Superset

	Single-arm pull-downs			Supernated curl		
Set and Rep:	1.	2.	3.	1.	2.	3.
Weight (kg):						

Superset

	Squat				Calf raise			
	1.	2.	3.	4.	1.	2.	3.	4
Sets								
Reps	30	30	30	30	15	15	15	15
Weight (kg)	20	20	20	20	20	20	20	20

Arm Haulers 4 × 30

Abs

½ sit-ups: 4 × 30
V-sit-ups: 4 × 30
Reverse curls: 4 × 30

My notes: I worked out this morning in the hotel's gym. I had only an hour to train because I had to go to Monaco, so I abbreviated everything.

Superset

	Squat				Calf raise			
	1.	2.	3.	4.	1.	2.	3.	4.
Sets								
Reps								
Weight (kg)								

Arm Haulers ✗

Abs

½ sit-ups: ✗
V-sit-ups: ✗
Reverse curls: ✗

Your notes:

WEEK 11 TESTS

Front view of me at the end of week 11.

Back view of me at the end of week 11.

MY WEEKLY TESTS

Weight (kg):   78.5
Height (cm):   175.5
BMI: 25.5
RHR: 39
BP: 135/44
Fat %:   12.5

Measurements (cm)
Neck: 38.10
Chest: 106.68
Arm: R 37.46   L 37.46
Navel: 78.28
Hips: 81.91
Thighs: R 61.59   L 61.59
Calves: R 40   L 40

YOUR WEEKLY TESTS

Weight (kg):
Height (cm):
BMI:
RHR:
BP:
Fat %:

Measurements (cm)
Neck:
Chest:
Arm: R   L
Navel:
Hips:
Thighs: R   L
Calves: R   L

WEEK **TWELVE** NUTRITION PLAN **WEEK 12**

WEEK 12 OVERVIEW

Day	Breakfast	Lunch	Dinner
1	Fresh fruit and seeds	Tuna salad	Jambalaya
2	Fruit smoothie 2	Smoked salmon pitta	Grilled sea bass with fresh vegetables
3	Muesli with fresh fruit	Sweet potato and bean salad	Vegetable Thai curry
4	Fruit porridge	Chicken salad pitta	Monkfish salad
5	Wheat biscuits or muesli with fruit	Butternut squash and coriander soup	Baked rainbow trout
6	Fruit salad	Mackerel salad	Lamb shanks
7	Omelette	Tuna and olive salad	Butternut squash and lentil stew

SHOPPING LIST **WEEK 12**

CARBOHYDRATES

75g brown basmati rice
50g wholegrain brown barley
1 bag of brown rice
400g kidney beans
525g lentils
25g millet seeds
250g of muesli
125g new potatoes
1 bag of pine nuts
400g pinto beans
560g porridge oats
3 potatoes
1 bag of sunflower seeds
1 bag pumpkin seeds
12 sweet potatoes
8 wholemeal or brown pitta breads
Wheat biscuits

DAIRY AND NON-DAIRY ALTERNATIVES

3 eggs
60g feta/goat's cheese
1880ml skimmed/soya/rice/oat milk
1.7kg soya yoghurt

FISH

8 anchovy fillets
225g fresh mackerel
600g monkfish tail
8 king size prawns
4 rainbow trout
4 sea bass fillets
4 pack of smoked salmon
4 small tins tuna
350g tuna steaks

MEAT

4 chicken breasts
4 chicken thighs
100g raw chorizo
100g raw garlic sausage
2kg lamb shank

400g lean ham

FRUIT

8 apples
2 apricots
10 bananas
1 lime
3 lemons
1 mango
2 oranges
2 peaches
1 large pineapple
1 small packet of raisins
1 punnet of raspberries
1 watermelon

VEGETABLES

3 avocados
100g baby corn
3 bags of baby spinach
1.4kg butternut squash
25g black olives
250g cherry tomatoes
5 carrots
4 celery sticks
3 courgettes
½ cucumber
175g French beans
3 green peppers
2 lettuces
50g mangetout
1 marrow
4 onions
115g baby plum tomatoes
1 red onion
5 red peppers
8 red tomatoes
100g rocket salad
1 shallot
100g sugar snap peas
10 spring onions
2 yellow peppers

HERBS

Basil

2 bay leaves
Black pepper
Coriander
Ground coriander
Ground cumin
Dill
1 garlic bulb
Fresh ginger
1 lemongrass stalk
Nutmeg
Oregano
Paprika
Parsley
1 red chilli
Rosemary
Turmeric

OTHER

Balsamic vinegar
Chicken stock
400ml coconut milk
Cold-pressed extra virgin olive oil
Dijon mustard
Plain flour
400g tinned plum tomatoes
Vegetable stock
115ml white wine
White wine vinegar

SNACKS

Fruit
Wholegrain crispbread crackers
Flat breads
Small bowl of muesli
Yoghurt/soya yoghurt
Nuts (cashew, pine or occasionally mixed nuts)
Soya nuts
Seeds (pumpkin or sunflower)

FRUIT DRINKS

1 carton fruit juice

RECIPES **WEEK 12** DAY 1

BREAKFAST FRESH FRUIT AND SEEDS

See page 82

LUNCH TUNA SALAD

See page 131

DINNER JAMBALAYA

4 skinless, boneless chicken thighs, halved

1 tablespoon flour

1 onion, peeled and finely chopped

½ red pepper, deseeded and chopped

½ green pepper, deseeded and chopped

50g wholegrain brown barley, soaked in boiling water and drained

230g tinned chopped tomatoes

500ml chicken stock

75g brown basmati rice

1 tablespoon olive oil

8 king size prawns, peeled

100g raw garlic sausage, roughly chopped and lightly dry-fried

100g raw chorizo, roughly chopped and lightly dry-fried

1 clove garlic, peeled and finely chopped

1 teaspoon fresh thyme leaves

1 red chilli, deseeded and roughly chopped

25g millet seeds, dry-fried until they 'pop'

1. Dust the chicken in the flour.
2. Heat the olive oil in a large non-stick frying pan and add the onion, garlic, red and green pepper, thyme and chilli to the pan and cook over medium heat until onion is soft.
3. Add the barley, tomatoes, chicken stock and bring to boil.
4. Add the chicken and sausages, lower the heat and stir in the rice and millet.
5. Cover and cook for 20 minutes or until the rice is almost tender.
6. Remove the lid and simmer for a further 10 minutes.
7. Stir in the prawns and cook for a further 5 minutes.
8. Serve on warm plates.

RECIPES **WEEK 12** DAY 2

BREAKFAST FRUIT SMOOTHIE 2   *See page 152*

LUNCH SMOKED SALMON PITTA   *See page 80*

DINNER GRILLED SEA BASS WITH FRESH VEGETABLES

4 fillets sea bass (150g each)

300g tinned lentils, drained and rinsed (try and use fresh lentils if you have time)

Broccoli and other green vegetables

For the marinade:

3 garlic cloves, peeled and crushed

2 tablespoon fresh parsley, chopped

2 tablespoon water

Black pepper

3 teaspoons dried oregano

4 teaspoons olive oil

4 tablespoons lemon juice

1. To make the marinade, mix the oregano, garlic, olive oil, lemon juice, black pepper, water and parsley together.
2. Wash the fish fillet and pat dry with kitchen towel. Then place on plate and spoon over half the marinade. Cover and refrigerate for 1–2 hours.
3. Preheat the grill to high.
4. Grill the fillet skin-side down for 5–6 minutes until just cooked through – the flesh should be white.
5. Meanwhile, warm the lentils with the marinade.
6. Spoon on to warm plates and place the sea bass on top.
7. Serve with fresh vegetables.

Lunch for tomorrow:
SWEET POTATO AND BEAN SALAD
Consider preparing the eggs and sweet potatoes in advance.

RECIPES **WEEK 12** DAY 3

BREAKFAST MUESLI WITH FRESH FRUIT

See page 80

LUNCH SWEET POTATO AND BEAN SALAD

See page 199

DINNER VEGETABLE THAI CURRY

400ml tin coconut milk

½ teaspoon ground coriander

½ teaspoon ground cumin

2cm fresh ginger, peeled and sliced

1 stalk of lemon grass, cut into 2cm pieces

100g sugar snap peas

1 red pepper, deseeded and sliced

1 yellow pepper, deseeded and sliced

100g baby corn, halved lengthways

2 courgettes, trimmed and chopped

2 spring onions, trimmed and finely sliced

Basil leaves to garnish

Brown rice

1 Heat coconut milk in a wok or large frying pan over a high heat.
2 Add ground coriander, ground cumin, ginger and lemon grass, and cook for 2–3 minutes.
3 Add the peas, peppers, baby corn and courgettes, and cook for a further 3–4 minutes or until vegetables are just cooked.
4 Garnish with spring onions and basil.
5 Serve with brown rice.

Lunch for tomorrow:
CHICKEN SALAD PITTA
Consider preparing chicken in advance (refrigerate overnight).

RECIPES **WEEK 12** DAY 4

BREAKFAST FRUIT PORRIDGE   *See page 81*

LUNCH CHICKEN SALAD PITTA   *See page 120*

DINNER MONKFISH SALAD

600g monkfish tail, washed with membrane removed

1 tablespoon olive oil

2 teaspoons rosemary, chopped

6 plum tomatoes

For the salad:

2 teaspoons olive oil

2 tablespoons pine nuts

1 garlic clove, peeled and sliced

450g baby spinach

2 tablespoons raisins

1 lemon, juice of

1 Preheat the oven to 220°C (425°F). Mix the olive oil and the rosemary in a small bowl, season with pepper and lightly coat the fish with this mixture.
2 Place the fish in a roasting tin with the tomatoes and bake in the oven for 20 minutes or until the fish is firm and white.
3 Meanwhile, heat the olive oil in a large frying pan, add the pine nuts and garlic, and cook until golden.
4 Add the spinach leaves, raisins and lemon juice a handful at a time.
5 Cut the fish from either side of the central bone.
6 Serve with the salad and cooking juices.

Lunch for tomorrow:
BUTTERNUT SQUASH AND CORIANDER SOUP
Consider preparing in advance (refrigerate overnight).

RECIPES **WEEK 12** DAY 5

BREAKFAST WHEAT BISCUITS OR MUESLI WITH FRUIT   *See page 84*

LUNCH BUTTERNUT SQUASH AND CORIANDER SOUP   *See page 88*

DINNER BAKED RAINBOW TROUT

4 rainbow trout, gutted

2 oranges, sliced with skin on

2.5cm fresh ginger, cut into slices

3 sweet potatoes, cut into small chunks

1 marrow, remove skin and cut into small chunks

2 garlic cloves, crushed

40g goat's/mature cheddar cheese

3 teaspoons dried basil

1 tablespoon olive oil

Salad leaves

For the dressing:

1 tablespoon fresh dill, finely chopped

250g plain soya/plain yoghurt

1 garlic clove, crushed

1 teaspoon balsamic vinegar

1 Preheat oven to 190°C (375°F).
2 Place the sweet potatoes, marrow, garlic and dried basil in a large baking dish and drizzle with olive oil.
3 Bake for 30–40 minutes or until cooked.
4 Add the cheese in the last 5–8 minutes.
5 Meanwhile, prepare the dressing by mixing all the dressing ingredients in a small bowl, then place in refrigerator.
6 Preheat the grill to medium.
7 Place two orange slices in each trout and sprinkle the ginger evenly between the fish.
8 Grill the fish for 12–14 minutes, turning occasionally.
9 Arrange the grilled trout on a bed of salad with the sweet potatoes and marrow.
10 Drizzle with the dressing and serve.

RECIPES **WEEK 12** DAY 6

BREAKFAST FRUIT SALAD   *See page 85*

LUNCH MACKEREL SALAD   *See page 88*

DINNER LAMB SHANKS

2 tablespoons olive oil

2kg lamb shanks on the bone

2 onions, chopped

1 celery stick

115ml white wine

675ml chicken stock

2 cloves garlic

2 bay leaves

2 tablespoons parsley

1 tablespoon lemon zest

Vegetables of your choice and new potatoes

1 Preheat oven to 160°C (325°F).
2 Heat a large heavy-based saucepan over a high heat.
3 Coat the lamb shanks with olive oil and cook in saucepan, turning occasionally, for 10 minutes or until well browned, then remove to a plate.
4 Add the garlic, onion and celery to the pan and cook for 5 minutes, or until soft.
5 Next add the wine, stock, lemon zest, parsley and bay leaves and bring to the boil.
6 Gently place the lamb shanks in a casserole dish and add the mixture from the pan.
7 Cover with foil and cook in oven for 1–2 hours, or until meat begins to fall off the bone.
8 Garnish with parsley and serve with steamed vegetables and new potatoes.

RECIPES WEEK 12 DAY 7

BREAKFAST OMELETTE   *See page 88*

LUNCH TUNA AND OLIVE SALAD   *See page 81*

DINNER BUTTERNUT SQUASH AND LENTIL STEW

225g lentils

2 onions, peeled and finely chopped

750ml vegetable stock

3 carrots, peeled and chopped

½ butternut squash, peeled, deseeded and chopped

1 sweet potato, peeled and chopped

3 small white potatoes, peeled and chopped

1 celery stalk, trimmed and chopped

50g frozen or fresh peas

1 Soak the lentils in cold water for 20 minutes, rinse and drain.
2 Bring the vegetable stock to the boil in a large saucepan.
3 Next, add the onions, lentils, carrots, squash, sweet potato and white potatoes and bring back to boil.
4 Lower the heat and simmer for 10–20 minutes.
5 Add the celery and simmer for a further 5 minutes.
6 Add the peas and simmer for a couple more minutes.
7 Serve in bowls.

TRAINING DIARY **WEEK 12**

WEEK 12 OVERVIEW
Day 1: CV – Run
Day 2: PT – Upper body
Day 3: CV – Cycle; Weights – Upper body;
      CV – Cycle
Day 4: CV – Run PT
Day 5: Weights – Upper body
Day 6: CV – Walk
Day 7: Tests

MY DIARY

Day 1 (Monday)
Got back early in the morning, so did my tests straight away as this still counts as my Sunday test day. I managed to fit a run in before spending the rest of the day with Alison and her family.
Tiredness 5
Stress 5
Sleep 6 hours

Day 2 (Tuesday)
It now feels like my final week and I'm really looking forward to it. I have been looking through the pictures and I just want to see what 12 weeks can do for me. I also have a lovely tan from being away on holiday, but again I'm peeling.
Tiredness 3
Stress 3
Sleep 6 hours 30 minutes

Day 3 (Wednesday)
Did some cycling and weight training today, and I'm feeling really good.
Tiredness 3
Stress 2
Sleep 5 hours 40 minutes

Day 4 (Thursday)
I'm starting to let my body and mind chill out for Sunday's test day, but that doesn't mean I'm stopping training, so I trained in the morning before going to work.
Tiredness 4
Stress 3
Sleep 5 hours 30 minutes

Day 5 (Friday)
I have a general all-over ache from this week's training. Today was my last weight training session before finishing, so I decided to do an all over session to make me feel good for Sunday.
Tiredness 3
Stress 2
Sleep 7 hours

Day 6 (Saturday)
I walked today with Alison, mainly to spend some quality time with her. My older brother came down to see the difference in me – he was shocked and very impressed. I had the day off with them both and just prepared for tomorrow, although I did manage to fit in one more lymphatic massage to take all my excess fluid out and leave me looking in good shape.
Tiredness 2
Stress 2
Sleep 8 hours

Day 7 (Sunday)
Test day. I went and saw my family and had a meal to celebrate. I can't believe the 12 weeks is over – you will notice that I have had good times and bad times, but as long as you keep mentally strong, with the right determination and your goal in mind, then all of this can happen to you.
Tiredness 2
Stress 3
Sleep 7 hours

TRAINING SESSION **WEEK 12** DAY 1

MY TRAINING SESSION

AM Rest

PM **Training session** CV – Run

Time trained 5.00–5.25 p.m.

Session time 25 minutes

RPE 10/10

WORKOUT
Run – 4 miles
Actual distance: 3.05 miles
Time: 20.30 minutes
Average Pace: 6.50 m/m

My notes: I went for a quick 3 mile run, I was exhausted.

YOUR TRAINING SESSION

AM

PM **Training session** CV – Run

Time trained

Session time

RPE   /10

WORKOUT
Run – 4 miles
Actual distance: miles
Time: minutes
Average Pace: m/m

Your notes:

TRAINING SESSION **WEEK 12** DAY 2

MY TRAINING SESSION

AM Rest

PM **Training session** PT – Upper body

Time trained 5.55–7.00 p.m.

Session time 1 hour 05 minutes

RPE 7/10

YOUR TRAINING SESSION

AM

PM **Training session** PT – Upper body

Time trained

Session time

RPE   /10

WORKOUT
No rest in between sets and reps

Bench press
10 × 100kg
20 × 70kg
30 × 50kg

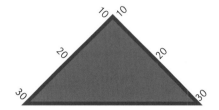

Incline press
10 × 100kg
20 × 70kg
30 × 50kg

Military press
10 × 55kg
20 × 40kg
30 × 20kg

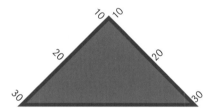

7-way kettle bell raises 1 × 10 reps

Arm haulers 3 × 75

Push-ups 5 × 40
Abs
½ sit-ups: 4 × 20
Reverse crunch: 4 × 20
Reverse curl: 4 × 20

My notes: I was trying to hit the areas I thought needed a little improvement.

WORKOUT
No rest in between sets and reps

Bench press
×   kg
×   kg
×   kg

Incline press
×   kg
×   kg
×   kg

Military press
×   kg
×   kg
×   kg

7-way kettle bell raises ×   reps

Arm haulers ×

Push-ups ×
Abs
½ sit-ups: ×
Reverse crunch: ×
Reverse curl: ×

Your notes:

TRAINING SESSION **WEEK 12** DAY 3

MY TRAINING SESSION

AM Training session CV – Cycle

Time trained 8.15–8.35 a.m.

Session time 20 minutes

RPE 8/10

PM Training session Weights – Upper body

Time trained 6.00–7.00 p.m.

Session time 1 hour

RPE 8/10

PM Training session CV – Cycle

Time trained 7.10–7.28 p.m.

Session time 18 minutes

RPE 9/10

YOUR TRAINING SESSION

AM **Training session** CV – Cycle

Time trained

Session time

RPE /10

PM **Training session** Weights – Upper body

Time trained

Session time

RPE /10

PM **Training session** CV – Cycle

Time trained

Session time

RPE /10

WORKOUT

Cycle – 10 miles
Actual distance: 8.2 miles

Weights – Upper body
Warm up on both exercises for 20 reps before beginning supersets.

Supersets

	Bench press			Pec fly		
Set and Rep	1. 30	2. 30	3. 30	1. 10	2. 10	3. 10
Weight (kg)	45	45	45	8	8	8

WORKOUT

Cycle – 10 miles
Actual distance: miles

Weights – Upper body

Supersets

	Bench press			Pec fly		
Set and Rep:	1.	2.	3.	1.	2.	3.
Weight (kg):						

	Incline press			Incline fly				Incline press			Incline fly		
Set and Rep	1. 30	2. 30	3. 30	1. 10	2. 10	3. 10	Set and Rep:	1.	2.	3.	1.	2.	3.
Weight (kg)	45	45	45	8	8	8	Weight (kg):						

	Bent-over row			Single arm cable row				Bent-over row			Single arm cable row		
Set and Rep	1. 30	2. 30	3. 30	1. 30	2. 30	3. 30	Set and Rep:	1.	2.	3.	1.	2.	3.
Weight (kg)	45	45	45	8	8	8	Weight (kg):						

	Bent-over lat raise			Arm haulers				Bent-over lat raise			Arm haulers		
Set and Rep	1. 10	2. 10	3. 10	1. 30	2. 30	3. 30	Set and Rep:	1.	2.	3.	1.	2.	3.
Weight (kg)	8	8	8				Weight (kg):						

	Upright rows			Lat raise				Upright rows			Lat raise		
Set and Rep	1. 10	2. 10	3. 10	1. 20	2. 20	3. 20	Set and Rep:	1.	2.	3.	1.	2.	3.
Weight (kg)	45	45	45	8	8	8	Weight (kg):						

Cycle – 10 miles
Actual distance: 8.2 miles

My notes: today I trained with a friend. This made me late to get to my parents for dinner, so I had to cycle as fast as possible to make up time.

Cycle – 10 miles
Actual distance:　　　　miles

Your notes:

TRAINING SESSION **WEEK 12** DAY 4

MY TRAINING SESSION

AM Training session CV – Run PT

Time trained 8.10–8.45 a.m.

Session time 35 minutes

RPE 7/10

PM Rest

YOUR TRAINING SESSION

AM Training session CV – Run PT

Time trained

Session time

RPE /10

PM

WORKOUT
Run PT
Actual distance: 4.32 miles

Run approximately 0.75 miles between the fitness stations. All exercises are 1 set of 100 reps. I broke the 100 reps into 5 × 20 reps, unless marked AIOH (all in one hit) which means I completed all 100 reps without stopping.

Run 1 mile to station 1 Dips: × 100
Press-ups decline: × 100

Run to station 2 Pull-ups: × 100
½ sit-ups: × 100
Sit-ups: × 100

Run to station 3 Reverse curls: × 100
Arm haulers: × 100

Run to station 4 Calf raises: × 100 AIOH
Squats: × 100 AIOH

Run 1 mile to finish

My notes: I trained in the morning before going to work. I only had a bit of time so I put 100 per cent into all the exercises with the smallest amount of rest between sets (roughly less than 30 seconds).

WORKOUT
Run PT
Actual distance: miles

Run 1 mile to station 1 Dips: ×
Press-ups decline: ×

Run to station 2 Pull-ups: ×
½ sit-ups: ×
Sit-ups: ×

Run to station 3 Reverse curls: ×
Arm haulers: ×

Run to station 4 Calf raises: ×   AIOH
Squats: ×   AIOH

Run 1 mile to finish

Your notes:

TRAINING SESSION **WEEK 12** DAY 5

MY TRAINING SESSION

AM Rest

PM Training session Weights – Upper body

Time trained 6.15–7.40 p.m.

Session time 1 hour 25 minutes

RPE 7/10

YOUR TRAINING SESSION

AM

PM Training session Weights – Upper body

Time trained

Session time

RPE   /10

WORKOUT

Bench press

1 × 20 warm-up – with just Olympic bar

Set and Rep:	1. 10	2. 10	3. 10	4. 7	5. 6
Weight (kg):	40	80	110	115	120

Warm-up on both exercises × 20 reps

Superset

	Incline fly		Morey squeeze (upper)	
Set and Rep:	1. 10	2. 10	1. 20	2. 20
Weight (lb)	55	55	25	25

Superset

	Arnold press		Lat raise	
Sets and Reps	1. 10	2. 10	1. 20	2. 20
Weight (lb)	35	35	25	25

Superset

	Regular pull-ups		Single arm row	
Sets and Reps	1. 20	2. 20	1. 10	2. 10
Weight (lb)			90	90

Superset

	Dips		Rope triceps press-downs	
Sets and Reps	1. 30	2. 30	1. 10	2. 10
Weight (kg)			20	20

Superset

	Hammer curl		Arm curl	
Sets and Reps	1. 10	2. 10	1. 20	2. 20
Weight (lb)	35	35	25	25

My notes: I wanted to lift as much as possible for my bench press, and I managed to achieve six good reps with 120kg. With the rest of the workout I had no rest between the sets and exercises. I completed the 1st set on both the superset exercises and then went straight back and complete the 2nd set.

WORKOUT

Bench press

1 × 20 warm-up – with just Olympic bar

Set and Rep:	1.	2.	3.	4.	5.
Weight (kg):					

Superset

	Incline fly		Morey squeeze (upper)	
Set and Rep:	1.	2.	1.	2.
Weight (kg)				

Superset

	Arnold press		Lat raise	
Set and Rep:	1.	2.	1.	2.
Weight (kg)				

Superset

	Regular pull-ups		Single arm row	
Set and Rep:	1.	2.	1.	2.
Weight (kg)				

Superset

	Dips		Rope triceps press-downs	
Set and Rep:	1.	2.	1.	2.
Weight (kg)				

Superset

	Hammer curl		Arm curl	
Set and Rep:	1.	2.	1.	2.
Weight (kg)				

Your notes:

TRAINING SESSION **WEEK 12** DAY 6

MY TRAINING SESSION

AM Training session CV – Walk

Time trained 10.00–10.45 a.m.

Session time 45 minutes

RPE 1/10

PM Rest

WORKOUT
Walk – 3 miles
Actual distance: 3.05 miles
Time: 45 minutes
Average pace: 15 m/m

My notes: I just wanted to take it easy before the big day tomorrow with all of my tests. I hope you have done as well as me with your results for tomorrow, if not better.

YOUR TRAINING SESSION

PM Training session CV – Walk

Time trained

Session time

RPE /10

PM

WORKOUT
Walk – 3 miles
Actual distance: miles
Time: minutes
Average pace: m/m

Your notes:

WEEK 12 HEALTH CHECK

MY RESULTS

Statistics	Weight (kg): 78
	Height (cm): 175.5
Health tests	BMI: 25.3
	RHR: 37
	BP: 127/44
	Fat (%): 11.9
	Glucose: 4.9
	Cholesterol: 3.9
	Lung function: 700
Measurements (cm)	Neck: 38.10
	Chest: 106.68
	Arms: R: 38.10 L: 38.19
	Navel: 78.19
	Hips: 81.28
	Thighs: R: 61.59 L: 61.59
	Calves: R: 40.64 L: 40.64
Calliper test (mm)	Biceps: 2
	Triceps: 6
	Waist: 7
	Subscapularis: 8
	Total: 23
	Calliper fat (%): 9.7
Fitness tests	Bleep test (level): 13.4
Maximum reps in one minute	Push-ups: 88
	½ sit-ups: 101
	Squats: 89
	Dips: 91
	Max pull-ups: 42
One rep maximum weight training (kg)	Squats: 137.5
	Bench press: 130
	Military press: 72.5
	Deadlifts: 140

YOUR RESULTS

Statistics	Weight (kg):
	Height (cm):
Health tests	BMI:
	RHR:
	BP: /
	Fat (%):
	Glucose:
	Cholesterol:
	Lung function:
Measurements (cm)	Neck:
	Chest:
	Arms: R: L:
	Navel:
	Hips:
	Thighs: R: L:
	Calves: R: L:
Calliper test (mm)	Biceps:
	Triceps:
	Waist:
	Subscapularis:
	Total:
	Calliper fat (%):
Fitness tests	Bleep test (level):
Maximum reps in one minute	Push-ups:
	½ sit-ups:
	Squats:
	Dips:
	Max pull-ups:
One rep maximum weight training (kg)	Squats:
	Bench press:
	Military press:
	Deadlifts:

BODYBUILDING POSES

Make sure you take a photo of yourself,
front and back and in the bodybuilding poses.

Front view of me at the end of
week 12.

Abdominal pose

Rear double biceps

Back view of me at the end of
week 12.

Front lat spread

Lat spread

THE FINAL RESULTS (INCREASES AND DECREASES)

MY RESULTS

Statistics	Weight (kg): −9.5
	Height (cm): 175.5
Health tests	BMI: −2.8
	RHR: −42
	BP: −6/48
	Fat (%): −9
	Glucose: −1.0
	Cholesterol: −2.0
	Lung function: +100
Measurements (cm)	Neck: −2.54
	Chest: +7.62
	Arms: R: +3.81 L: +3.20
	Navel: −9.52
	Hips: −8.89
	Thighs: R: + 1.27 L: + 2.54
	Calves: R: same L: + 1.27
Calliper test (mm)	Biceps: −4
	Triceps: −2
	Waist: −8
	Subscapularis: −4
	Total: −18
	Calliper fat (%): −6.9
Fitness tests	Bleep test (level): gained over 2.5 levels
Maximum reps in one minute	Push-ups: +29
	½ sit-ups: +4
	Squats: +37
	Dips: +36
	Max pull-ups: +30
One rep maximum weight training (kg)	Squats: +27.5
	Bench press: +30
	Military press: +12.5
	Deadlifts: +20

YOUR RESULTS

Statistics	Weight (kg):
	Height (cm):
Health tests	BMI:
	RHR:
	BP: /
	Fat (%):
	Glucose:
	Cholesterol:
	Lung function:
Measurements (cm)	Neck:
	Chest:
	Arms: R: L:
	Navel:
	Hips:
	Thighs: R: L:
	Calves: R: L:
Calliper test (mm)	Biceps:
	Triceps:
	Waist:
	Subscapularis:
	Total:
	Calliper fat (%):
Fitness tests	Bleep test (level):
Maximum reps in one minute	Push-ups:
	½ sit-ups:
	Squats:
	Dips:
	Max pull-ups:
One rep maximum weight training (kg)	Squats:
	Bench press:
	Military press:
	Deadlifts:

THE NEW YOU CAN TAKE YOU ANYWHERE

Here I am (left photo) with two extra stone on me and not looking my best. On the right is me at the end of the 12-week programme. It's amazing what 12 weeks can do.

Finally, the photos below are of me in preparation for and during a professional photograph shoot taken by one of the world's leading men's magazines. If I can do this, imagine what you can do.

ANATOMY AND EXERCISES

07

CHEST MUSCLES

Outer pectoral major

Upper pectoral major

Inner pectoral major

Lower pectoral major

Serratus anterior

Inner pectoral

MIDDLE, OUTER AND INNER PECTORALS

BENCH PRESS (COMPOUND)

Purpose
To build mass, strength and density in the pectorals, anterior deltoids and triceps.

Action
- Lie on the bench, with your feet flat on the floor.
- Your grip should be wider than shoulder width, with an overhand grip.
- Raise bar off rack.
- Lower the bar under control, until the bar comes in alignment with or slightly below your nipples.
- Press the bar back up until arms are almost locked out.

PEC FLY

Purpose
To enhance the mass of the pectoralis major.

Action
- Lie on the bench, with your feet flat on the floor.
- Hold dumbbells above your chest, palms facing each other.
- Lower weights out and down, with your elbows slightly bent, until your pectorals are fully stretched.
- Return to the starting position following the same large arch, while squeezing your chest.
- Once at the top, keep a small gap between the weights and flex the pectorals to maximise full contraction.

DUMBBELL BENCH PRESS

Purpose

Develops mass on the outer and middle pectorals.

Action

- Lie on the bench, with your feet flat on the floor.
- Grasp the dumbbells in your hands, and hold the weights above your chest, with your palms facing forwards
- Lower the dumbbells to your outer pectorals as far as you can go while feeling a stretch.
- Press the weight back up, squeezing your chest, until your arms are almost locked out and keeping a small gap between the weights.

>>

STRAIGHT ARM PULL-OVERS (DUMBBELLS)

Purpose

This develops the pectoralis major, as well as expanding your ribcage.

Action

- Lie on the bench, with your feet flat on the floor.
- Hold dumbbell with both of your hands.
- Hold the weight above your chest with a small bend in your elbow.
- Lower the weight behind your head as far as you can go, until your pectorals and rib cage are fully stretched.
- Return to the starting position following the same large arch, while squeezing your chest.

<<

<<

CABLE CROSS-OVER

Purpose

To develop the inner portion of the pectoralis major and pectoralis minor.

Action

- While holding the pulley handles, step slightly forwards.
- Extend your arms to your sides and lean forwards from your waist.
- With your palms facing each other and your elbows slightly bent, bring your hands together following the same arch as pec flies.
- Contract the pectorals when your hands are in the centre, but keep going until your hands have crossed each other so that one hand is wrapped underneath the bar and the other is wrapped over the top of the bar. Alternate per repetition.

PRESS-UP

Purpose

To develop the pectoralis major and triceps.

Action

- Lie flat on the floor face down.
- Place your hands on the floor slightly wider than your shoulders, pointing up towards your head and in line with your nipples.
- Place your toes on to the floor, and raise your legs and hips off of the floor.
- Keep your back nice and straight until you have finished your set.
- Extend your arms by pushing into the floor, without arching your back.
- Lower back down to the starting position, not allowing your knees or legs to come into contact with the floor.

¾ PRESS-UP

Use if you are unable to perform a regular press-up.

Action

- Lie flat on the floor face down.
- Place your hands on the floor slightly wider than your shoulders, pointing up towards your head and in line with your nipples.
- Place your toes and the tops of your knees on to the floor.
- Raise your hips and upper body off of the floor, keeping your back nice and straight.
- Extend your arms by pushing into the floor, without arching your back.
- Lower back down to the starting position.

WIDE PRESS-UPS

Purpose

To develop the outer part of pectoralis major.

Action

- Lie flat on the floor face down.
- Place your hands on the floor wider than shoulder-width apart, pointing away from your body at 45° and in line with your nipples.
- Place your toes on to the floor and raise your legs and hips off of the floor.
- Extend your arms by pushing into the floor, without arching your back.
- Lower back down to the starting position, not allowing your knees or legs to come into contact with the floor.

DIAMOND PRESS-UPS

Purpose

To develop the inner part of pectoralis major, and a lot of emphasis on your triceps.

Action

- Lie flat on the floor face down.
- Place your hands in a triangular shape, index fingers and thumbs touching, in front of your body in alignment with your lower pectorals.
- Place your toes on to the floor, and raise your legs and hips off the floor.
- Lean slightly over your hands and extend your arms by pushing into the floor, without arching your back.
- Squeeze your chest at the top to get the most out of your inner pectorals.
- Lower back down to the starting position, not allowing your knees or legs to come into contact with the floor.

LOWER PECTORALS

DECLINE BENCH PRESS

Purpose
To develop mass, strength and density in the lower pectorals.

Action
- Place the bench at a decline angle of 30°.
- Lie on the bench, with your feet around the bench pads.
- Your grip should be wider than shoulder width, with an overhand grip.
- Raise bar off rack.
- Lower the bar under control until the bar comes into alignment with or slightly below your nipples.
- Press the bar back up until arms are almost locked out.

MOREY SQUEEZE (LOWER)

Purpose
To work the lower and middle pectorals.

Action
- Extend one arm to your side while supporting yourself with either a bench or weight.
- Draw your hands up and inwards until the weight is roughly in alignment with the opposite nipple, while keeping a slight bend in your elbow.
- Flex your lower pectoral to get the full benefit.
- Following the same arch bring the weight back down to your side.

UPPER PECTORALS

INCLINE PRESS

Purpose
To develop and build mass and strength of the upper pectorals, anterior deltoids and triceps.

Action
- Place the bench at an incline angle of 45°.
- Lie on the bench, with your feet flat on the floor.
- Your grip should be wider than shoulder width, with an overhand grip.
- Raise the bar off the rack.
- Lower the bar under control to your upper pectorals, just below your collarbone.
- Press the bar back up until arms are almost locked out.

INCLINE DUMBBELL PRESS

Purpose
To develop mass on the middle and upper pectorals.

Action
- Place the bench at an incline angle of 45°.
- Lie on the bench, with your feet flat on the floor.
- Grasp the dumbbells in your hands and hold the weights above your upper chest, with your palms facing forwards.
- Lower the dumbbells to your outer pectorals as far as you can go while feeling a stretch, in line with your upper pectorals, just below your collarbone.
- Press the weight back up until arms are almost locked out, while keeping a small gap between the weights.

INCLINE FLY

Purpose
To build mass on the upper pectorals.

Action
- Place bench at an incline angle of 45°.
- Lie on the bench, with your feet flat on the floor.
- Hold dumbbells above your chest, with palms facing each other.
- Lower weights out and down, with your elbows slightly bent, until your pectorals are fully stretched.
- Return to the starting position following the same large arch, while squeezing your chest muscles.
- Once at the top, keep a small gap between the weights and flex the pectorals to maximise full contraction.

MOREY SQUEEZE (UPPER)

Purpose
To develop and define the upper and slight middle pectorals.

Action
- Extend one arm to your side while supporting yourself with either a bench or weight.
- Draw your hands up and inwards until the weight is roughly in alignment with the opposite shoulder, while keeping a slight bend in your elbow.
- Flex your upper pectoral to get the full benefit.
- Following the same arch, bring the weight back down to your side.

SERRATUS ANTERIOR

ROPE PULLS

Purpose

To work and develop the serratus anterior. Your abdominals and lats are also brought into use.

Action

- Hold on to the upper pulley and kneel on the floor.
- Keep your arms extended above your head, curl your body forwards and down, pulling with your lats.
- Keep pulling until your elbows have touched your sides, and curl your head towards your knees.
- Uncurl and come back up to the start, feeling a stretch in your lats.

>>

PULL-OVERS

Purpose

Works the lower lats and serratus anterior.

Action

- Lie on the bench with your arms bent and weight on your chest.
- Move the bar over your head slowly, while keeping your arms bent, until you feel your lats stretch (the weight should never touch the floor).

<<

BACK MUSCLES

Rotator cuff
Infraspinatus,
teres major

Latissimus dorsi

Trapezius
upper

Trapezius
lower

Rhomboids
under
trapezius

Outer
latissimus
dorsi

Lower
latissimus
dorsi

Erector
spinae

FULL SWEEP AND DEVELOPMENT OF THE BACK

REGULAR PULL-UPS >>

Purpose
To create the full sweep of the lats
and develop the teres major.

Action
- Hold the chin bar, with your
hands over shoulder-width apart
and with an overhand grip.
- Hang from the bar so that your
feet are not touching the ground
and your arms are straight.
- Pull your body up, trying to reach the top of your chest to the bar.
- At the top, hold yourself for a brief moment.
- Lower your body to the start, with your arms straight.

REVERSE PULL-UPS >>

Purpose

To develop your lats, teres major and biceps.

Action

- Hold the chin bar, with your hands shoulder-width apart and with an underhand grip.
- Hang from the bar so your feet are not touching the ground and your arms are straight.
- Pull your body up, trying to reach the top of your chest to the bar.
- At the top, hold yourself for a brief moment.
- Lower your body to the start, with your arms straight.

DEADLIFTS (COMPOUND)

Purpose

An overall power exercise that involves more than one muscle group and works the lower back.

Action

- Place the barbell on the floor in front of you.
- With your legs hip-width apart, bend your knees and lean forwards from the hips to grasp the bar.
- Grasp the bar with a medium to wide grip, one hand in an overhand grip and the other in an underhand grip.
- Keep your abdominal muscles contracted and your back in a neutral position to protect from the strain.
- Lift by driving with your legs first, and then straighten up until you are standing upright.
- Push your chest out and shoulders back.
- Lower the weight by bending your knees and leaning forwards from the waist.
- Touch the weight just above the floor to begin your next rep.

SINGLE ARM ROW

Purpose
Isolates the lats on one side, as well as developing and defining the centre of your back.

Action
- Grasp the dumbbell in one hand, with your palm facing inwards.
- Place the opposite knee and hand on the bench, keeping a neutral back.
- Begin with the weight hanging by your side at full stretch, allowing your body to tilt towards the weight.
- Raise your upper arm and elbow as high as possible, next to your body.
- Lower under control, and repeat until you have finished your reps, before repeating with the other arm.

>>

LOW PULL/SEATED ROW

Purpose
To bulk and develop the thickness of the back and lower lats.

Action
- Sit facing the machine, with your feet on the pads and knees slightly bent.
- Extend your arms and lean slightly forwards, feeling a stretch in your lats, even when the weight stack is at the bottom.
- Pull the handle towards your upper abdominals, while squeezing your shoulder blades back and down.
- Your chest should stick out, sitting upright and not leaning back.
- Control the weight back to the start, again feeling the stretch in your lats.

<<

UPPER BACK DEVELOPMENT

BENT-OVER ROWS

Purpose
To develop and thicken the upper back.

Action
- Stand with your feet hip-width apart and your knees slightly bent.
- Grasp the bar with a wide and overhand grip.
- Bend forwards so your upper body is between 45° and parallel with the floor.
- Allow the bar to hang in front of your shin bones, with your head and back straight.
- Lift the bar up towards the upper abdominals/diaphragm.
- Keep your elbows close to your body, and feel your back work.
- Lower the bar back down to the start.

T-BAR ROW (IMPROVISED)

Purpose
Thickens your outer and upper back.

Action
- Straddle the bar, keeping your feet hip-width apart.
- Slightly bend your knees, bend forwards to 45° keeping a flat back, and take hold of the weight.
- Without changing position, lift the weight up to your lower pectoral before lowering it back down to get a full stretch.
- Remember, if you feel it in your lower back or legs you will need to take off some plates to isolate the upper back.

REVERSE SHRUG

Purpose

To strengthen your lower trapezius. Excellent for office workers.

Action

- Place the weight on a squat rack.
- Face away from the bar, then back into and grasp the bar with your palms facing away (overhand grip).
- To begin, lift bar, rotate your shoulder blades back and down in one motion and squeeze, while sticking your chest out.
- Remember, the movement is very small and you should not feel anything in your upper traps.
- Return by allowing your arms to rotate forwards.

WIDEN YOUR BACK/LATS

WIDE PULL-UPS

Purpose

To widen your upper back and enhance the full sweep of the lats.

Action

- Hold the chin bar with your hands as wide as practical to perform the pull-up, with an overhand grip.
- Hang from the bar so your feet are not touching the ground and your arms are straight.
- Pull your body up, trying to reach the top of your chest to the bar.
- At the top, hold yourself for a brief moment.
- Lower your body to the start and with your arms straight.

MOUNTAIN CLIMBER PULL-UPS

Purpose
To widen and lengthen your lats, and develop the serratus anterior.

Action
- Hold the chin bar with your hands facing each other, one in front of the other and with an overhand grip.
- Hang from the bar so your feet are not touching the ground and your arms are straight.
- Pull your body up so your head goes to the side of the bar and your shoulder reaches the bar.
- At the top, hold yourself for a brief moment.
- Lower your body to the start, with your arms straight.
- To train the other side, swap your hands so the other hand is in front.

LAT PULL-DOWNS

Purpose
To develop the bulk of your back and widen your upper lats.

Action
- Hold the bar with a wide overhand grip.
- Sit on the bench, with your knees/feet under the supports.
- While sticking out your chest and leaning backwards 5–10°, pull the bar down, squeezing your shoulder blades back and down while leading with your elbows until the bar is at the top of your chest in alignment with your collar bone.
- Allow your arms to extend back to the start under control before repeating.

DEVELOPING LOWER LATS AND LOWER BACK

CLOSE PULL-UPS

Purpose

To widen and lengthen your lower lats, and develop the serratus anterior.

Action

- Hold the chin bar with your hands close together and with an overhand grip.
- Hang from the bar so your feet are not touching the ground and your arms are straight.
- Pull your body up, trying to reach the top of your chest to the bar.
- At the top, hold yourself for a brief moment.
- Lower your body back to the start, with your arms straight.

CLOSE GRIP PULL-DOWNS

Purpose

To develop the lower lats.

Action

- Hold the bar with a close overhand grip.
- Sit on the bench, with your knees/feet under the supports.
- While puffing out your chest, pull the bar down with your elbows pulling back to the top of your chest.
- Allow your arms to extend back to the start under control.

SINGLE ARM CABLE ROW

Purpose

To develop your lower lats using the full range of motion.

Action

- Use a floor-level pulley.
- Take hold of the handle and stand in a balanced position with the opposite leg forwards.
- Begin with your arm fully outstretched in front of you, palm down.
- Pull the handle while twisting your hand to face up.
- Pull your elbow back as far as possible.
- Extend your arm back out in front while twisting your hand palm down to feel the stretch in your lats.

PULL-OVERS

Purpose

Works the lower lats and serratus anterior.

Action

- Lie on the bench with your arms bent and weight on your chest.
- Move the bar over your head slowly, keeping your arms bent, until you feel your lats stretch (the weight should never touch the floor).
- Raise the weight back to your chest, while concentrating on your lats

LOWER BACK

DORSAL RAISE

Purpose

To strengthen the spinal erectors (lower back).

Action

- Lie face down, with your whole body touching the floor.
- Arm placement varies. Easy – arms by your side; medium – fingers on temples; hard – arms straight out in front.
- Raise your chest off the floor using your lower back.
- Remember to keep your hips and feet on the floor at all times.
- Lower yourself back down and repeat.

SHOULDER MUSCLES

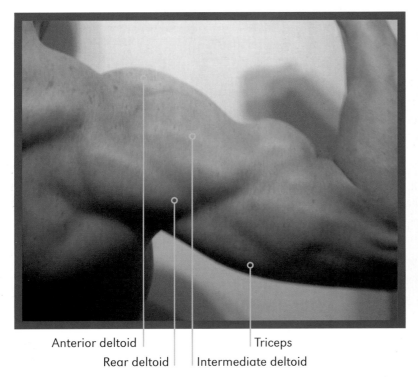

Anterior deltoid

Rear deltoid

Triceps

Intermediate deltoid

Triceps Deltoid Biceps

ANTERIOR AND MEDIAL DELTOIDS

MILITARY PRESS

Purpose
Bulks and thickens the anterior and medial deltoids.

Action
- Perform from a standing or seated position (seated is more challenging).
- Grasp the bar with an overhand grip, and hold it in alignment with your collar bone/shoulder with elbows tucked in.
- Press the bar straight up overhead, until your arms are straight but not locked out.
- Lower the weight under control to the start position.

>>

ARNOLD PRESS

>>

Purpose

Develops the anterior and medial deltoids.

Action

- From a standing or seated position, hold the dumbbells with your palms turned towards you.
- As you begin to press-up, turn your arm and palms out in a smooth motion, while pushing your arms up until they are almost locked out.
- Once at the top pause for a second.
- Return by lowering the weight and rotating your palms back to the starting position.

<<

DUMBBELL PRESS

Purpose

To develop anterior and medial deltoids, and give more range of motion than the military press.

Action

- Perform from a standing or seated position (seated is more challenging).
- Grasp the dumbbell, with palms facing forwards and in alignment with your collar bone/shoulder with elbows tucked in.
- Press the dumbbells straight up overhead until the weights almost touch at the top, and with your arms straight but not locked out.
- Lower the weight under control to the start position.

UPRIGHT ROWS

Purpose

Develops separation between deltoids and pectorals. Works the upper trapezius and anterior deltoids, while strengthening your shoulder girdle.

Action

- Stand with your legs hip-width apart and grasp the bar with an overhand grip, with a gap of 10–20cm between your hands.
- Lift the bar up towards your chin.
- Pause and then lower under control keeping the weight close to your body.

>>

FRONT ARM RAISES

Purpose
To develop the anterior deltoid.

Action
- Perform from a standing or seated position.
- Grasp the weight in your hand, and lift one hand up in a large arch until the weight is higher than your head.
- Make sure the weight passes in front of your face to maximise the anterior deltoid.
- Lower the weight smoothly and under control.

LATERAL RAISE

Purpose
To develop the medial deltoids.

Action
- Hold the dumbbells in each hand, with the weights together and in front of you, and palms facing each other.
- Feet should be hip-width apart, and arms slightly bent and leaning partially forwards.
- Raise the weights up and out, leading with your elbow.
- Bring the weight slightly higher than your shoulder, while making sure the weight doesn't go higher than the elbow.
- Lower slowly and keeping control until the weight touches at the bottom, before the next repetition.

REAR DELTOID

BENT-OVER LAT RAISE

Purpose
To develop the rear deltoids.

>>

Action
- Hold the dumbbells in each hand, with the weights together and to the front of you, and palms facing each other.
- Feet should be hip-width apart, and arms slightly bent.
- Lean forwards at the waist to about 45°, while keeping a straight back.
- Lift the weights to either side of your head, remembering not to allow them to go behind your shoulders.
- To accentuate the rear deltoids, twist your hands so the thumb ends up lower than your little finger.
- Lower the weight under control and repeat.

ARM HAULERS

Purpose
To work all of your deltoids, especially the rear deltoid.

Action
- Lie face down, with your back slightly arched.
- Start with your arm straight and above your head.
- Bring your arms directly down to your side.
- Remember, your arms or hands should not to touch the ground.
- Bring your arms back up to the top and repeat, always keeping your feet on the ground.

ALL-OVER SHOULDER

7-WAY KETTLE BELL RAISES

Purpose
To work all of your deltoids.

Action
- Hold the kettle bell in one hand, palm facing you.
- Hold the weight to your side with a slight bend in your elbow.
1. Using the weight as a momentum, raise your arm diagonally to the front, across your body, so the weight comes into alignment with the opposing shoulder.
2. Front arm raise.
3. Arm raise to the front, which is 45° out to your side. Allow the weight to swing all the way through behind you.
4. Lat raise.
5. Arm raise behind you, 45° out to your side of the body. Raise as high as comfortable, with your palm facing diagonally forwards towards your body. Remember to swing the weight slightly in front of you.
6. Rear lat raise, palms facing forwards.
7. With your palm facing back and towards your body, raise the weight diagonally behind you, squeezing your shoulder blade, and trying to feel your rear deltoid.

<<

ARMS: BICEPS MUSCLES

Biceps   Anterior   Pectoral major
          deltoid

Biceps   Triceps

BICEPS SIZE AND SHAPE

ARM CURL (OLYMPIC BAR)

Purpose

To develop the mass and overall size of the biceps.

Action

- Stand with your back straight, and your feet hip-width apart.
- Grasp the bar with an underhand grip, with your hands shoulder-width apart.
- Let the bar hang in front of you with your arms straight.
- Curl the bar in an arch that goes up and out, bringing it as high as is comfortable.
- Keep your elbows close and pivoted to the side of your body.
- Contract the biceps at the top before lowering the weight back down under control to the start.
- A narrow grip mainly works the outer biceps (long head).
- A wide grip mainly works the inner biceps (short head).

DUMBBELL ARM CURL

Purpose

Allows you to concentrate on the development of the individual biceps.

Action

- Stand with your back straight and your feet hip-width apart.
- Grasp the dumbbells with an underhand grip, with your hands shoulder-width apart facing away from the body.
- Let the dumbbells hang in front of you, with your arms straight.
- Curl the dumbbells in an arch that goes up and out, bringing it as high as is comfortable.
- Keep your elbows close and pivoted to the side of your body.
- Contract the biceps at the top before lowering the weight back down under control to the start.

SUPERNATED CURL

Purpose

Develops the size and shape of the biceps.

Action

- Stand with your back straight and your feet hip-width apart.
- Grasp the dumbbell with an underhand grip, with your hands facing your body shoulder-width apart.
- Curl one dumbbell in an arch, while twisting your wrist so your palm ends up facing you.
- Keep your elbows close and pivoted to the side of your body.
- Contract the biceps at the top before lowering and twisting the weight back down under control to the start.

HEIGHT OF BICEPS

CABLE ARM CURL

Purpose
Develops the shape and height of biceps.

Action
- Stand with your back straight and your feet hip-width apart.
- Grasp the bar from the lower pulley, with an underhand grip and your hands shoulder-width apart, facing away from the body.
- Allow your biceps to stretch, while being straight.
- Curl the bar in an arch that goes up and out, bringing it as high as is comfortable.
- Keep your elbows close and pivoted to the side of your body.
- Contract the biceps at the top before lowering the weight back down under control to the start.

>>

<<

INCLINE DUMBBELL CURLS

Purpose
Develops the mass of the biceps and gives you a greater range of motion.

Action
- Place the bench at an incline angle of 45°.
- Lie on the bench, with your feet flat on the floor.
- Grasp the dumbbells with an underhand grip, and your palms facing in towards your body.
- Keep your arms extended and your elbows forwards.
- Curl the weights up to your deltoid in an arch, while twisting your wrists so your palms end up facing you.
- Contract the biceps at the top before lowering the weights back down under control to the start.

CONCENTRATED CURL

>>

Purpose
Develops the height/peak of the biceps.

Action
- Stand or sit with your back straight and your feet shoulder-width apart.
- Lean forwards from your hip, and grasp the dumbbell with an underhand grip.
- Rest your elbow against your inner thigh while keeping your arm straight.
- With your free hand, rest it on your opposing knee.
- Curl the dumbbell in an arch towards your deltoid, not your chest.
- To increase the peak of your biceps, twist your hand so your little finger goes higher than your thumb.
- Contract the biceps at the top before lowering the weight back down under control to the start.

HAMMER CURL

>>

Purpose
This is the best exercise to develop the brachioradialis. Also develops your brachialis, along with your biceps.

Action
- Stand with your back straight and your feet hip-width apart.
- Grasp the dumbbells with an underhand grip, with your hands shoulder-width apart facing towards your body.
- Keeping your palms facing your body, curl the dumbbells in an arch which goes up and out, bring it as high as comfortable.
- Keep your elbows close and pivoted to the side of your body.
- Flex at the top before lowering the weight back down under control to the start.

PREACHER CURL

Purpose
To develop the lower part of your biceps.

Action
- Stand or sit, with your back straight and your feet hip-width apart.
- Grasp the bar/dumbbell with an underhand grip, with your hands shoulder-width apart.
- Rest yourself on to the support, with your chest against the bench.
- Let the bar/dumbbell hang in front, with your arms straight.
- Curl the bar/dumbbell in an arch that goes up and out, bringing it as high as is comfortable.
- Contract the biceps at the top before lowering the weight back down under control to the start.

<<

ARMS: TRICEPS AND FOREARM MUSCLES

Deltoids   Triceps   Triceps

DEVELOP ALL THREE HEADS

TRICEPS PRESS-DOWNS

Purpose
To develop the whole triceps.

>>

Action
- Stand facing the machine, with your feet shoulder-width apart and back straight.
- Take hold of the bar from the upper pulley, with an overhand grip and your hands 10–20cm apart.
- Press the bar down towards your thighs as far as possible, while keeping your elbows tucked into your sides.
- Contract your triceps at the bottom, and then allow the bar to come back up to the top.
- Change the attachments and hand placements to work all the triceps heads.
- Medial head of triceps – reverse grip triceps press-down with bar.
- Lateral head of triceps – rope triceps press-down.
- Long head of triceps – overhead press with back to machine.

TRICEPS KICKBACKS

Purpose

To develop the whole triceps.

Action

- Hold one dumbbell with an overhand grip.
- Stand with one foot in front of the other.
- Place your free hand on your knee, or rest the free hand on a bench with the same hand and leg on the bench for stability.
- Keeping your back straight and leaning forwards from your waist, bend your elbow and raise it back to about shoulder height.
- Allow the weight to hang below your elbow.
- Keeping your elbow tucked into your side, raise the weight so your arm seems to be parallel with the floor.
- Squeeze at the top for the full benefits before allowing the weight to come back to the start.
- Make sure your upper arm doesn't move during the action.

SKULL CRUSHER

Purpose

To develop the triceps.

Action

- Lie on the bench, with your head all the way down to the end.
- Grasp the bar with an overhand grip, approximately 12–13cm apart.
- Press the weight up above your pectorals until your arms are straight out in front of you.
- Keeping your elbows stationary, lower the bar past your forehead, and then pause before pressing it straight back up, but this time with the weight just above your head when fully extended. This keeps constant tension on your triceps.

BENCH DIPS

Purpose

To develop the thickness of the triceps.

Action

- Suspend yourself between two benches or chairs, with your feet on one and the heels of your hands on the other.
- Your hands should be shoulder-width apart and facing forwards.

- Keeping your arms straight, lower yourself to the floor while keeping upright and your back close to the bench.
- Once at the bottom press back up, and once at the top contract your triceps as much as possible to get the full benefits.

EMPHASIS ON LATERAL HEAD

ROPE TRICEPS PRESS-DOWN

Purpose
To develop all three heads of the triceps, especially the lateral head.

Action
- Stand facing the machine, with your feet shoulder-width apart and back straight.
- Take hold of the rope from the upper pulley, with your hands in front of you and facing each other.
- Pull the rope down and out past your thighs as far as possible, while keeping your elbows tucked into your side.
- Squeeze your triceps at the bottom as hard as possible, and then allow the bar to come back up to the top, bringing your arms back to the front.

SINGLE ARM PULL-DOWNS

Purpose
Develops the horseshoe shape, and isolates the triceps (especially the lateral head).

Action
- Stand facing the machine, with your feet shoulder-width apart and back straight.
- Take hold of the handle from the upper pulley, holding the handle with a reverse underhand grip.
- Extend the handle down as far as possible towards your thigh, while keeping your elbows tucked into your side.
- Squeeze your triceps at the bottom as hard as possible, and then allow the bar to come back up to the top, bringing your arm back to the front.

OVERHEAD TRICEPS EXTENSIONS (ONE ARM)

Purpose
Develops and separates the three heads of the triceps. Has a little more emphasis on the long head triceps.

Action
* Sit or stand, with your feet shoulder-width apart, and back straight.
* Take hold of the dumbbell with one hand and extend it above your head.
* Keeping your elbow stationary and close to your head.
* Lower the dumbbell behind your head until you feel a stretch in your triceps.
* Press the weight back up to the start.
* Squeeze your triceps at the top as hard as possible and then repeat.

<<

OVERHEAD TRICEPS EXTENSIONS (TWO HANDS)

>>

Purpose
Develops and separates the three heads of the triceps. Has a little more emphasis on the long head triceps.

Action
* Sit or stand, with your feet shoulder-width apart, and back straight.
* Take hold of the dumbbell with both hands and extend it above your head.
* Keeping your elbows stationary and close to your head.
* Lower the dumbbell behind your head until you feel a stretch in your triceps.
* Press the weight back up to the start.
* Squeeze your triceps at the top as hard as possible and then repeat.

LEG MUSCLES

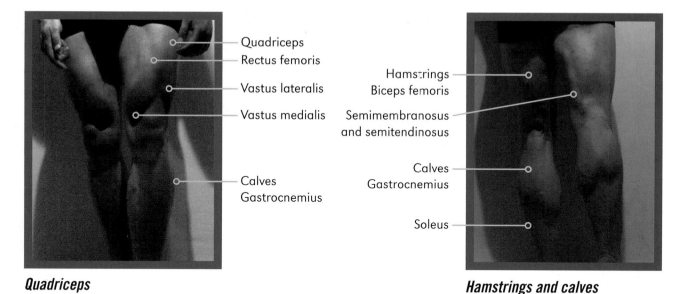

Quadriceps

Hamstrings and calves

QUADRICEPS

SQUATS (COMPOUND)

Purpose

To develop mass and strength in all four heads of the quadriceps, and strengthen your glutes.

Action

- With the barbell resting on a rack, stand under the bar and place it on to the trapezius.
- Hold on to the bar, with your hands at a comfortable width and in an overhand position.
- Lift the bar off the rack and step forwards, clear of the rack.
- Your feet should be shoulder-width apart, and toes naturally facing slightly outwards.
- Keeping your head up and back straight, bend at the knees and forwards from the hips.
- Try to remember to stick your glutes out on the way down, to help keep a straight back (as if you are about to sit down).
- When your thighs are horizontal with the floor or slightly below, push yourself back up to the starting position through your feet.
- Finish by walking the bar back on to the rack.
- Medial heads – feet facing out in squats.
- Lateral heads – narrow-stance squats.
- Medial heads and inner thighs – wide-stance squats.

>>

SQUAT JUMPS

Purpose

To build muscular endurance and develop all four quadriceps and glutes.

Action

- Hold the dumbbells down by your side, with your hands in an overhand position.
- Your feet should be shoulder-width apart, and toes naturally facing slightly outwards.
- Keeping your head up and back straight, bend at the knees and forwards from the hips.
- Try to remember to stick your glutes out on the way down, to help keep a straight back.
- When your thighs are horizontal with the floor or slightly below, push yourself back up and through into a jump, keeping the weights besides you.
- As soon as you land start the repetition.

\>\>

BOSU SQUATS

Purpose

To build muscular endurance, balance and develop all four quadriceps and glutes.

Action

- Hold the dumbbells down by your side, with your hands in an overhand position.
- Stand on the bosu (up or down), with your feet shoulder-width apart (or whatever the bosu allows), and your toes naturally facing slightly outwards.
- Keeping your head up and back straight, bend at the knees and forwards from the hips.
- Try to remember to stick your glutes out on the way down, to help keep a straight back.
- When your thighs are horizontal with the floor or slightly below, push yourself back up to the starting position.

SINGLE SIDE SQUATS

Purpose
To develop the quadriceps.

Action
- Hold the dumbbells down by your side, with your hands in an overhand position.
- Stand with one leg up on a step box and the other flat on the floor.
- Your feet should be slightly wider than shoulder-width apart, and your toes naturally facing slightly outwards.
- Keeping your head up and back straight, bend at the knees and forwards from the hips.
- Allow all your weight to be on the leg that is flat on the floor, while the other is for balance.
- Try to remember to stick your glutes out on the way down, to help keep a straight back.
- When your thigh is horizontal with the floor or slightly below, push yourself back up to the start.

<<

FRONT SQUATS

Purpose
To develop the quadriceps and the lateral quadriceps.

>>

Action
- With the barbell resting on a rack, face the barbell and keep the bar above your arms.
- With your arms in front, cross your arms and cross your elbows.
- Grasp the bar so it sits across the top of your shoulders and chest.
- Lift the bar off the rack and step backwards, clear of the rack.
- Stand with your feet shoulder-width apart, and toes naturally facing slightly outwards.
- Keeping your head up and back straight, bend at the knees and forwards from the hips.
- Try to remember to stick your glutes out on the way down, to help keep a straight back.
- When your thighs are horizontal with the floor or slightly below, push yourself back up to the starting position through your feet.
- Finish by walking the bar back on to the rack.

SISSY SQUATS

Purpose
To isolate the lower quadriceps.

Action
- Stand upright, holding on to either a bench or rack.
- Keep your feet hip-width apart, bend your knees, and raise yourself on your toes.
- Allow your body to slowly drop towards the floor, pushing your hips and knees forwards.
- At the same time you should be tilting your head and shoulders back to keep balance.
- Go as low as is comfortable, before straightening your legs and coming back to the start.
- In the standing position, flex your quadriceps as hard as possible before doing your next repetition.

GLUTES AND QUADS

LUNGES (STATIC)

Purpose
Develops the glutes and quadriceps.

Action
- With the barbell resting on a rack, stand under the bar and place it on to the trapezius.
- Hold on to the bar with your hands at a comfortable width and in an overhand position.
- Lift the bar off the rack and step forwards, clear of the rack.
- Keeping your trunk straight, head up and chest out, take a lunge forwards with your leading leg.
- The lunge should be long enough so that your trailing leg is almost straight.
- From this starting position bend your front knee, ensuring your front knee remains behind your toes and your trailing knee goes towards the ground.
- Push yourself back up with your leading leg.
- From this static position, repeat for the number of repetitions with this leg, and then swap to your other leg.

BOSU LUNGE (STATIC) >>

Purpose

Develops the quadriceps and glutes, while improving balance.

Action

- Perform with or without a dumbbell (hold on to the dumbbells with palms facing your body).
- Keeping your trunk straight, head up and chest out, take a lunge forwards with your leading leg on the bosu, either way round.
- The lunge should be long enough so that your trailing leg is almost straight.
- From this starting position bend your front knee, ensuring your front knee remains behind your toes and your trailing knee goes towards the ground.
- Push yourself back up with your leading leg.
- From this static position, repeat for the number of repetitions with this one leg, and then swap to your other leg.

LUNGES >>

Purpose

Develops the glutes and quadriceps.

Action

- With the barbell resting on a rack, stand under the bar and place it on to the trapezius. If using dumbbells, hold the weight next to your body, with palms facing in.
- Hold on to the bar with your hands at a comfortable width, and in an overhand position.
- Lift bar off the rack and step forwards, clear of the rack.
- Keeping your trunk straight, head up and chest out, take a lunge forwards with your leading leg.
- The lunge should be long enough so that your trailing leg is almost straight.
- Bend your front knee, ensuring your leading knee remains behind your toes and your trailing knee goes towards the ground.
- Push yourself back up to the standing position with your leading leg, so that your feet go hip-width apart
- Repeat for the number of repetitions with the same leg, and then swap to your other leg.

STANDING GLUTE EXTENSIONS

Purpose
To isolate and firm the glutes.

Action
- Stand facing a wall, with both arms on the wall for support.
- Keeping your pelvis forwards, extend your leg backwards from your hips with your knee slightly bent.
- Squeeze your gluteus muscle as hard as possible at the top of the movement, then return to the start.

>>

GLUTE EXTENSIONS

Purpose
To isolate and firm the glutes.

Action
- While on all fours, kneel on one leg and bring the other towards your chest, while leaning on your hands with your arms extended.
- Extend your leg backwards from your hips, leading with your foot.
- You can have your leg straight, but I prefer to keep my knee bent to hit the glutes even more.
- Squeeze at the top of the movement to get the most out of the glute extension, before returning your leg all the way through to your chest again.
- Repeat for the specific number of repetitions, before changing to your other leg.

DIRTY DOGS

Purpose
To develop your gluteus medius and deeper gluteal muscles.

Action
- While on all fours, kneel on one leg and lean on your hands with your arms extended.
- Keep your leg in the bent position, and raise your leg up to your side from your hip.
- You should squeeze at the top and feel the burn on the side of your gluteals.
- Lower back down and repeat.

STANDING HIP ABDUCTION

Purpose
To develop your gluteus medius and deeper gluteal muscles.

Action
- Stand facing a wall, with both arms on the wall for support.
- Keeping your pelvis forwards, extend your leg backwards at a 45° angle from your hips, and with your knee slightly bent.
- Squeeze your gluteal muscles as hard as possible at the top of the movement, then return to the start.

HAMSTRINGS

STIFF LEG DEADLIFTS >>

Purpose
To develop the hamstrings.

Action
- Place the barbell on the floor in front of you.
- With legs hip-width apart, bend your knees and lean forwards from the hips to grasp the bar.
- Grasp the bar with a medium to wide grip, using an overhand grip with one hand and an underhand grip with the other.
- Keep your abdominal muscles contracted and back in a neutral position to protect from the strain.
- Lift by driving with your legs first, and then straighten up until you are standing upright.
- Push your chest out and shoulders back.
- Lower the weight by leaning forwards from the hips, keeping your legs as straight as comfortable, but making sure your knees are not locked out.
- At the bottom of the movement you should feel a stretch in your hamstrings before returning to the top. Repeat for the sets and reps specified.

CALVES

STANDING CALF RAISES

Purpose
To develop the mass of the calves.

Action
- Stand either on the floor or on a block.
- With the barbell at knee height on the rack, take hold of it with an underhand grip for one hand and an overhand grip for the other.
- If on a block, lower your heels to the floor, stretching your calves.
- Keeping your knees slightly bent, raise up on to your tip-toes and flex as much as possible.
- Pause for a second, then return under control either to the floor or, if on a block, all the way down to a big stretch.
- Medial head of the gastrocnemius – toes turned out.
- Lateral head of the gastrocnemius – toes turned in.

<<

ABDOMINAL MUSCLES

Rectus abdominis upper and lower

Obliques

ABDOMINALS

FULL SIT-UPS

Purpose
To work the rectus abdominis and hip flexors.

Action

- Lie on your back with your knees bent and together, and your feet, back and head flat on the floor.
- Hand position varies the difficulty: easy – arms across your body; intermediate – fingers by your temples; hard – arms straight and directly above your head.
- Curl your body off the ground with your head first, then shoulders, upper back, and finally your lower back.
- All the time you should be thinking of sucking your navel (belly button) into the ground.
- Once at the top pause, then return back to the start, but this time don't pause at the bottom.

<<

V-SIT-UPS

Purpose

To work your upper and lower abdominals.

Action

- Lie on your back with your legs at a 35° angle, off the floor and together.
- Make sure your back and head are flat on the floor, and your arms straight out overhead.
- Simultaneously curl your upper body and lower body off the ground together.
- Upper body – raise your head first then shoulders, and finally your upper back and your arms following above your head.
- Lower body – raise your legs from 35° to approximately 80°, while keeping them straight and together.
- All the time you should be thinking of sucking your navel (belly button) into the ground.
- Once at the top pause, then return back to the start, but this time don't pause at the bottom.

INCLINE SIT-UPS

Purpose

These put greater emphasis on your abdominals and hip flexors than a regular full sit-up.

Action

- Place the bench at a decline of approximately 45°.
- Hook your feet under the pads, and lie on your back with your knees bent and together if possible.
- Position your feet, back and head flat on the floor.
- Hand position varies the difficulty: easy – arms across your body; intermediate – fingers by your temples; hard – arms straight and directly above your head.
- Curl your body off the ground with your head first, then shoulders, upper back, and finally your lower back.
- All the time you should be thinking of sucking your navel (belly button) into the ground.
- Once at the top pause, then return back to the start, but this time don't pause at the bottom.

PLANK

Purpose

To strengthen the core muscles.

Action

- Lie face down, supporting yourself on your forearms and toes.
- To start, raise your body off the ground so all your body weight is being placed on to your toes and forearms.
- Make sure your body is straight and flat and tighten your abdominals, obliques and lower back.
- Hold in this position for the time required, before returning back down.

UPPER ABDOMINALS

HALF SIT-UPS

Purpose

To work the upper abdominals.

Action

- Lie on your back with your knees bent and together.
- Feet, back and head flat on the floor.
- Hand position varies the difficulty: easy – arms across your body; intermediate – fingers by your temples; hard – arms straight and directly above your head.
- Curl your body off the ground with your head first, then shoulders, and finally your upper back.
- All the time you should be thinking of sucking your navel (belly button) into the ground.
- Once at the top pause, then return back to the start, but this time don't pause at the bottom.

CRUNCHES

Purpose

Emphasises the upper abdominals.

Action

- Lie on your back, legs either in the air or resting on a bench.
- Keep your knees bent and together, with your back and head flat on the floor.
- Hand position varies according to difficulty: easy – arms across your body; intermediate – fingers by your temples; hard – arms straight and directly above your head.

LOWER ABDOMINALS

REVERSE CRUNCH

Purpose

To strengthen and develop your lower abdominals.

Action

- Lie on your back with your legs in the air.
- Keep your knees bent and together, with your back and head flat on the floor.
- Place your hands by your side.
- Curl your lower back and glutes off the ground. All the time you should be thinking of sucking your navel (belly button) into the ground.
- Once your knees are by your chest pause, then return back to the start, but this time don't pause at the start.

LEG LEVERS

Purpose

To strengthen and develop your lower abdominals.

Action

- Lie on your back with your legs together and straight.
- Keeping your back and head flat on the floor, place your arms to your side for balance.
- Keeping your feet 10cm off the floor, raise your legs up and out in a wide arch up to 80°.
- All the time you should be thinking of sucking your navel (belly button) into the ground.
- Once at the top pause, then return slowly back to the start, but this time don't pause at the bottom.
- Note that when you lower your legs and your lower back starts to arch off the floor, it is at this point you raise your legs back up to top. This stops any involvement with your lower back.

REVERSE CURLS

Purpose
To strengthen your lower abdominals.

Action
- Lie on your back with your legs together and straight.
- Keeping your back and head flat on the floor, place your palms under your glutes/sacrum, face down making a triangular shape with your hands, with index fingers and thumbs touching.
- Raise your legs to start at a 90° angle in the air.
- Curl your lower abdominals, so your legs end up going up and towards you in a smooth diagonal motion.
- This is a small action – when you get it right you will feel a burning sensation from your navel (belly button) and below.
- All the time you should be thinking of sucking your navel (belly button) into the ground.
- Once at the top pause, then return slowly back to the start, but this time don't pause at the bottom.

OBLIQUES

OBLIQUE SIDE CRUNCHES

Purpose
To strengthen the obliques.

Action
- Lie on one side, with your upper body resting on the forearm and the lower body, hips, legs and feet in contact with the ground.
- Place your free hand either by your side or in front of you for balance.
- Raise your whole body off the ground, while supporting yourself on the side of your feet and forearm.
- Hold your body straight, almost like a side plank.
- Once in this position, raise your hip in the air by concentrating on contracting the oblique nearest the ground.
- Hold and flex, before lowering back down to the side plank position.

HEEL TAPS

Purpose
To work the obliques.

Action
- Lie on your back with your knees bent and together.
- Place your feet, back and head flat on the floor.
- Put your arms by your side and lift your head off the ground slightly.
- Crunch your body and arm towards one heel, squeezing your oblique.
- To complete a full repetition, move back to the centre, over to the other side, and back to the centre again.
- All the time you should be thinking of sucking your navel (belly button) into the ground.

JUMPING OBLIQUE TWISTS

Purpose
Tighten and work obliques

Action
- Start with your feet hip-width apart.
- Twist your lower torso to one side while trying to keep your upper body still.
- Twist your lower torso all the way round to the other side.

OTHER EXERCISES

BURPEES

Purpose

To condition and develop muscular endurance and strength in your whole body.

Action

- Start with your feet shoulder-width apart and ready to move into a squat position.
- Squat down and place your hands on the floor in front of you.
- Kick your feet back into a press-up position, while performing a regular press-up.
- On the way up from the press-up, immediately return to your feet in the squat position.
- Leap as high as possible, before returning back into the squat position for the next repetition.

SQUAT THRUSTS

Purpose
To build muscular endurance in your legs.

Action
- Start with your feet shoulder-width apart, and ready to move into a squat position.
- Squat down, and place your hands on the floor in front of you.
- Kick your feet back into a press-up position.
- While in this position, bring your knees up as high as you can towards your chest.
- Return your feet back out straight to the press-up position. This is one repetition.
- Repeat for the specified number of repetitions, before returning to your feet.

ALTERNATE SQUAT THRUSTS

Purpose
To build muscular endurance in your legs.

Action
- Start with your feet shoulder-width apart, and ready to move into a squat position.
- Squat down and place your hands on the floor in front of you.
- Kick your feet back into a press-up position.
- Stay in this position. Keep one leg out straight while you bring your other knee up as high as you can towards your chest.
- Then alternate your legs over, so the leg that was straight is now up by your chest and the other leg is out straight. Once both your knees have been up to your chest once, this counts as one repetition.
- Once you have finished the repetitions specified, return your feet out straight behind you and squat thrust up and on to your feet.

>>

FROG HOPS

>>

Purpose

To develop muscular strength and endurance in your lower legs.

Action

- Start from a squatting position, with your feet shoulder-width apart.
- Jump forwards as far and as high as you can, landing on both feet.
- Pause for a second, and then repeat for the specified number of repetitions.

JUMP OVERS

Purpose

To develop muscular strength and endurance in your lower legs.

Action

- Start with your feet hip-width apart, and next to a step box or an object approximately 45cm high.
- Jump over the object to the other side with your feet together and immediately back after touching the ground.
- Repeat for the specified number of repetitions.

<<

WIDE SQUAT THRUSTS

Purpose

To build muscular endurance in your adductors and abductors.

Action

- Start with your feet shoulder-width apart and ready to move into a squat position.
- Squat down and place your hands on the floor in front of you.
- Kick your feet back into a press-up position.
- While in this position, abduct your legs out to the side as far as possible, before adducting your feet together again.
- Repeat for the specified number of repetitions, before returning to you feet.

>>

STAR JUMPS

Purpose

Improves muscular endurance, fitness and coordination.

Action

- Stand with your feet shoulder-width apart, with your arms by your side.
- As you jump, raise your arms up to the side (shoulder height) and abduct your legs to the side as far as comfortable, then you will land in the position of a star.
- Jump back from that position to the start and repeat.

SPOTTY DOGS

Purpose

Improves muscular endurance, fitness and coordination.

Action

- Stand with one foot forwards (leading leg), with the same-side arm out in front of you at shoulder height.
- Jump into the air so you swap your leading leg and arms over, so your opposite leg is now out in front.

SKIPPING

Purpose

Improves fitness, coordination and rhythm.

Action

- Hold on to the handles at waist height and slightly in front of you.
- As you jump, try to rotate the rope by making small rotations from your forearms, and with a little help from your wrists.
- One turn of the rope and one bounce counts as one repetition.

STEP BOX EXERCISES

STEP-UPS

BOX JUMPS

If you find this too much on your joints, do down, down, up, up instead.

DOWN, DOWN, UP, UP

SIDE LUNGES

BACK LUNGES

BOXING EXERCISES

ALTERNATE PUNCHES >>

 << STRAIGHT PUNCHES

UPPER CUTS >>

 << WIDE PUNCHES

REVERSE PUNCHES >>

WEIGHT AND RUNNING CONVERSION CHARTS

WEIGHT CONVERSION CHART

Throughout the training sessions we have used kilograms and pounds. Use the weight conversion chart below to monitor and calculate the weight you have been lifting.

Kilograms (kg)	Pounds (lb)
1	2.2
5	11
10	22
15	33
20	44
25	55
30	66
40	88
50	110
60	132
70	154
80	176
90	198
100	220
110	242
120	264
130	286
140	308
150	330

MINUTE/MILE CONVERSION CHART

Use the following minute/mile conversation chart to see how long it takes you to run a certain distance. I have highlighted a good pace to be aiming for.

Miles	1	2	3	4	5	6	8	10
6	6	12	18	24	30	36	48	60
7	7	14	21	28	35	42	56	70
8	8	16	24	32	40	48	64	80
9	9	18	27	36	45	54	72	90
10	10	20	30	40	50	60	80	100
12	12	24	36	48	60	72	96	120
15	15	30	45	60	75	90	120	150

Minutes per mile

RELEASE THE PRESSURE

08

MASSAGE AND STRETCHING

Massage is one of the oldest and simplest forms of medical care used to ease pain and anxiety, and to promote good health. Massage therapy and stretching provides relaxation and relief to muscle strain and fatigue, and this contributes to our overall health and well-being.

The benefits of massage therapy are almost endless, and include physical, emotional and physiological improvements to the body.

During the 12-week programme it is worth considering having massages to help relieve muscular spasms and tension, aid in the breaking down of cellulite, boost the immune system and stimulate the lymphatic system.

MUSCULAR MASSAGE
Uses pressure or trigger points and essential oils to work with massage to eliminate pain patterns. This

approach ultimately brings balance between the musculoskeletal system and the nervous system.

LYMPHATIC MASSAGE
Features special pumping strokes and vibrations to enhance the flow of the lymphatic system. Lymph is a whitish coloured liquid that flows throughout the body inside lymph vessels, which collect waste and toxins that cannot be absorbed through the capillary blood vessels. The combined movement and pressure encourages the movement of lymphatic fluid. This helps the immune and lymph systems, plus any

other types of oedema, to return to full health and correct working order.

MYO STRETCHING ROUTINE

Throughout the 12-week programme I used the myo stretch, which is an hour-long stretching routine. The myo stretch encompasses and works the majority of the muscles within your body to ensure an increase in muscle strength and resistance.

There are multiple benefits to stretching, and it should not be overlooked in your daily health routine. When we stretch properly we:

- Increase our range of motion (ROM)
- Increase performance in training and exercise (power and strength)
- Improve posture
- Reduce fatigue within muscles
- Reduce any delayed onset of muscle soreness after training or exercise (DOMS)
- Develop body awareness
- Promote circulation
- Improve relaxation within tense and tight muscles
- Aids stress relief

HOW TO STRETCH CORRECTLY

There is no time limit to stretching, although do remember that less is best. The gentler you are with your stretching, the more you get out of the muscles. When you find the first part of tension in your stretch, you should feel a really small amount, as if you are just about to stretch. It should be nice and simple, and isolate the muscle you are trying to focus on without involving any others. Allow the muscle adequate time to relax and elongate (there is no time limit).

If you are bouncing in stretches, feeling sharp pain in the muscle being stretched, feeling muscle spasm or shake, or feeling a burning sensation, then you are probably stretching the muscle too hard, and most likely incorrectly. Remember, less is best.

There are different types of stretching that can improve flexibility and strength, and are an important element when creating harmony within your body.

Static stretching

This means performing a certain stretch without movement. This is when you find the first tension within the muscle and hold, without moving from that position. Once it has released, you can either move on to the next stretch or gently repeat the action.

Developmental stretching

This works in the same way at the static stretch. You find the first point of tension and hold it until the muscle relaxes and elongates. Once you feel no stretch, go slightly further into the stretch until you feel tension for the second time. Repeat up to four times.

Proprioceptive neuromuscular facilitation stretching (PNF)

An advanced stretching and flexibility technique that involves both the contraction and stretching of a muscle. This stretch is best performed with a professional or training partner, although some can be tried at home. Always remember to listen to your body and take note on how to perform the PNF correctly, and do not use the PNF stretch on muscles that are weak, elongated or overstretched.

To perform PNF stretching:

- Find the first bit of tension in the stretch and hold until the tension has elongated.
- Contract the same muscle that was being stretched for 20–40 per cent of your maximum effort.
- Hold the contraction of the muscle for 12 seconds.
- Release the contraction and allow the muscle to relax for a second.
- Now find the second stretch by going further until you find the tension again. You should have noticed a greater range before feeling the stretch.
- Again, allow the stretch to relax and elongate before repeating the process.
- You can repeat this process up to three times before coming out of the stretch.

MYO STRETCH

Developmental stretch for calf (gastrocnemius) muscles

- From a press-up position, move your hand closer to your feet while raising your hips into the air.
- With your feet together, use one foot for support with the other foot flat on the floor and your legs extended straight, but not completely locked out.
- Bend the leg that is for support.
- Move your hands closer until you feel a small stretch in the calf of the foot that is flat to the ground.
- Once the stretch has elongated, move your hands closer again to your feet, or you can push your heel into the floor. You should now be feeling a stretch in the middle part of your calf muscle.
- Without dropping the position, allow your hands to go back to the starting position and repeat for the other leg. You will also be working your upper body while in this position.
- Once you have completed the stretch on the other side, move your hands back to the start, keeping in the same position. You are now ready to perform the soleus stretch.

Developmental stretch for soleus muscles

- Stay in the position of the calf stretch – with your hands out in front of you and your hips in the air.
- With your feet together, use one for support and the other almost flat on the floor, legs bent at the knee.
- Move your hands closer until you feel a small stretch in the lower calf.
- Once the stretch has elongated, move your hands closer to your feet, or you can push your heel into the floor. You should be feeling a stretch on the lower calf towards your Achilles tendon.
- Without dropping the position, allow your hands to go back to the starting position and repeat for the other leg. You will also be working your upper body while in this position.
- Once you have completed the stretch on the other side, put both feet on the floor and go back down into the press-up position.
- Sit up and sit back on to your heels. You are now ready to move on to the lower back stretch.

Static stretch for the lower back

- While sitting on your heels, reach forwards from your hip with your hands out in front of you and let your head relax.
- You should be nice and relaxed, and you might be able to feel a stretch in your lower back and latissimus dorsi.

Developmental stretch for hip flexor stretch

This is a good stretch for a lordotic posture:

- Kneel on one foot.
- If you need to, hold on to an object to help keep balance.
- Lean slightly forwards so your weight is on the front foot.
- Push your hip out forwards.
- To get more of a stretch, lean your torso slightly back in the opposite direction. You should feel a stretch in the front of your hip (iliacus, psoas major and rectus femoris).
- From this position go straight into the PNF stretch on the same leg.

PNF stretch for hamstring muscles

This is a postural stretch for flat back/sway back:

- Kneel on one knee with your other leg out in front, so your foot is flat on the floor.
- Keep your back straight while leaning forwards to keep balance (you can either balance yourself with one or both arms down to the floor).
- Sit back on to your knee.
- Try to keep your leg out in front, with a small bend in your knee.
- Tilt your buttocks up in the air to feel more of a stretch. As long as you have the stretch in your hamstrings you can now perform a PNF stretch if your muscle requires it.
- Follow the rules for performing a PNF stretch (see page 341).
- While in the same position, and now that the first stretch has released, you can push your foot into the ground as if you were trying to curl your heel up to your bum. You should now feel the same muscle contract that was just being stretched (if you can't feel the contraction in your hamstring, try moving until you do feel it).
- Hold the contraction at 20 per cent of your maximum effort for 12 seconds.
- Relax for one second, and then move into the stretch for a second time.
- Perform the PNF stretch two or three times. You should feel a stretch in the back of your thigh/hamstring (semimembranosus, semitendinosus and biceps femoris).
- Sit back on to both of your heels.
- Now change legs and repeat these last two stretches.

Static stretch for the lower back

- While sitting on your heels, reach forwards from your hip with your hands out in front of you and let your head relax.
- You should be nice and relaxed, and you might be able to feel a stretch in your lower back and latissimus dorsi.
- Sit back up on to your heels.

Developmental stretch for quad with your knees bent

- While sitting on your heels, place your legs under your buttocks.
- Lean back, keeping your body weight on your arms.
- You should then be able to feel a stretch in the middle part of your quads.
- To feel more of a stretch, or to develop the stretch, move your hands further behind you or squeeze your glute muscles/push out your hips. You should be able to feel a stretch within the middle part of your quads (rectus femoris, vastus medialis, vastus lateralis and vastus intermedius).
- Roll over on to your front and lie face down.

PNF stretch for quad lying face down

This is a posture stretch for lordotic postures.

- Lie face down.
- Bring one foot up towards your buttock while holding on to it with the same-side arm.
- Pull the foot to your buttock to feel the stretch within the middle/upper part of the quad.
- As long as you have the stretch in your quads you can now perform a PNF stretch if your muscle requires it. Follow the rules for performing a PNF stretch (see page 341).

- While in the same position, and when the first stretch has released, you can push your leg out as if you are trying to straighten it. You should now feel the same muscle contract. (If you can't, try to move slightly until you feel the muscle contract.)
- Hold the contraction at 20 per cent of your maximum effort for 12 seconds.
- Relax for one second, and then move into the stretch for a second time.
- Perform the PNF stretch two or three times.
- You should be able to feel a stretch within the middle to upper portion of the quads (rectus femoris, vastus medialis, vastus lateralis and vastus intermedius).
- Once you have stretched your quad, swap your hands over so your opposite hand is on the leg being stretched.
- From this position, go straight into the static stretch for the quads on the same leg.

Static stretch for quad muscles lying down, opposite hand to opposite leg

- Lie face down.
- Bring one foot up towards your buttock, while holding on to it with the opposite arm.
- Pull the foot to your opposite buttock.
- Keep your hips on the ground. You should be able to feel a stretch on the outer part of the quad).
- Once you have finished stretching, move on to your other leg and repeat.
- Once you have finished your lying quad stretches you can relax for 1 or 2 minutes in this position.
- Roll on to your back and sit up for your hamstring stretch.
- Repeat these last two stretches on the other leg.

Developmental stretch for sitting hamstring muscles

This is a posture stretch for flat back or sway back.

- Place your arms on the ground beside you.
- Place both legs out in front of you.
- Sit with your back straight.
- Bend one knee enough so it falls to the side, while keeping your other leg straight.
- Lean forwards from the hip until you find a stretch in your hamstrings. You should now be able to feel a stretch within your hamstring muscles (semimembranosus, semitendinosus and biceps femoris).
- Once you have stretched one side, move on to the other side.
- When you have finished stretching your other leg, keep both legs out in front of you ready for the next stretch.

Developmental stretch for the wide leg adductor

- Sit with your legs straight out and wide in front of you (make sure it is as wide as is comfortable so that you don't feel a stretch on your hamstring muscles).
- Sit with a straight back.
- Lean forwards until you feel a stretch on your adductors. You should be able to feel the inside of your thighs/adductors (adductor longus, adductor brevis, adductor magnus and gracilis).
- Bring both feet into your groin, if possible with your feet together, to stretch adductors.

Developmental stretch for the sitting groin muscle

- Sit with your back straight.
- For support, hold on to your feet.
- Keep your feet together if possible, and allow your knees to drop out to the side.
- You should feel a stretch on the inside of your thighs. If not, bring your feet in towards your groin.
- You should be able to feel a stretch on the inside of your thighs/ adductors (adductor longus, adductor brevis , adductor magnus, gracilis and pectineus).
- Put both of your legs out in front of you and relax your body for one or two minutes.

Static stretch for sitting glute muscle extensions

Perform this stretch if you feel pain in your lower back.

- Sit with one leg out straight, and cross the other leg over your knee.
- Turn your shoulders around so your torso is facing away from your body.
- Place one arm on to your raised knee to help you rotate even further, and your other arm out behind you to support yourself. You should be able to feel a stretch in your glute muscles (gluteus maximus, gluteus medius and gluteus minimus), as well as tensor fasciae latae and piriformis.
- Swap your legs over to stretch your other side.
- Keep your leg crossed but relaxed. Roll on to your back to stretch your deeper glute muscles.
- Change your legs over and repeat the same stretch.

Developmental stretch for glute muscles

Perform this postural stretch when suffering from sciatica (caused by your piriformis being too tight).

- Lie on your back on the floor, face up.
- Cross one leg over the other.
- Start to bring your foot down towards your buttock.
- Grasp on to the thigh (hamstrings) just under the knee.
- Pull the leg up and towards your chest. You should be able to feel a stretch in your glute muscles (piriformis, deep glute muscles and gluteus maximus).
- Stretch the other side, then relax with your feet on the ground and your knees in the air.
- Bring both knees into your chest to stretch your lower back.
- Change your legs over and repeat the stretch on the other side.

Developmental stretch for the lower back while lying down
Perform this postural stretch if you have a lordotic posture.

- Lie on your back, face up.
- Hold on to the back of both of your thighs, just underneath the knees.
- Pull your knees towards your chest, allowing your buttocks to rise off the ground. You should be able to feel a stretch in your lower back and gluteus maximus.
- Once the stretch has released, drop your feet on to the floor with knees bent and relaxed.
- Drop legs flat to the floor for the next stretch.

Static stretch for the whole body

- Lie on your back and extend your legs out straight in front of you, and your arms out straight overhead.
- Lengthen your body as much as possible by pointing your toes and pushing your arms overhead. You should be able to feel a stretch in different places of the body (including your abs, serratus anterior and lattisimus dorsi).
- Once the stretch has relaxed, bring your arms out to your side for the next stretch.

Static stretch for lying roll over
- Lie on your back.
- Keep your arms out to your side and bring your knees up, with your feet on the floor.
- Allow your knees to drop to one side and try to relax your back and hips to get the best stretch. You should be able to feel a stretch in your lower back muscles and glute muscles.
- Bring your knee back up to the centre and drop to the other side.
- Stay on your back in a relaxed position, and relax for 2–3 minutes.
- Roll on to your front for the abdominal stretch.

Static stretch for the abdominal muscles

This is a postural stretch for a flat back.

- Lie face down on the floor.
- Keep your hands in front of you, about shoulder-width apart.
- Keep your hips, legs and feet flat on the ground.
- Raise your torso off the ground until your arms are almost straight, or you feel a stretch in your abdominals.
- Hold this stretch for no longer than 10 seconds.

Static stretch for the oblique muscles

- Lie on your side, keeping your body straight.
- Make sure the leg you're resting is touching the floor.
- With your forearm resting on the floor and your other arm in front of you for support, extend your resting arm out straight so your body weight is resting on your hand instead.
- You should now feel a stretch on your side and in your oblique muscles.
- Roll on to your front, and then on to the other side, to stretch your other obliques.
- Once you have stretched your other side, roll back on to your front for the cat stretch.

Static cat stretch

- Kneel on all fours.
- Let your head fall forwards and relax.
- Arch your back and draw in your belly button. You should be able to feel a stretch in your lower back.
- Relax from your stretch, and then sit back on your heels for another lower back stretch.

Static stretch for the lower back

- While sitting on your heels, reach forwards from your hip with your hands out in front of you and let your head relax. You should be nice and relaxed, and you might be able to feel a stretch in your lower back and latissimus dorsi.
- Stay in this position, you're ready to get on to the next stretch.

Development lat stretch on the floor

- Sitting on your heels, reach forwards with your hands.
- Place one arm across your body with it resting on the floor.
- Use your fingers to walk your arm diagonally away from your body to feel a stretch in your latissimus dorsi.
- Keep walking your fingers out to get a developmental stretch.
- Bring your arm back to the centre, and then swap over to the other side.

Static stretch for the biceps muscles

- Kneel on all fours.
- Turn your arms so the insides of your forearms are facing away from you, and your fingers are pointing at you.
- Keep your arms straight, and sit back towards your heels.
- Try not to put too much body weight on to your arms. You should feel a stretch on the front of the top of your arms (the biceps, and possibly on your wrist flexors).
- Sit back up on to your heels, and relax for 2–3 minutes.

Static stretch for the triceps muscles

- Sit on your heels.
- Place one hand up and behind your head, with your elbow pointing upwards.
- With your other hand (depending on your flexibility), either pull the elbow down from the top, or you can push the elbow from the front. You should be able to feel a stretch on the back of your upper arm (triceps).
- Now stand up for the final stretches – you can move around to get the blood flowing around your muscles.
- Follow the next stretches one after the other while standing.

Static stretch for wrist flexor muscles

- With one hand, hold on to the fingers of your other hand and straighten your arm so your forearm is facing upwards.
- Pull your fingers/hand towards your body. You should be able to feel a stretch on the inside of your forearm.
- Repeat this stretch on your other hand.

Static stretch for the wrist extensor muscles

- With one hand, hold on to the opposite fingers/hand and straighten your arm so your forearm is facing down.
- Pull your fingers/hand towards your body. You should be able to feel a stretch on the back of your forearm.
- Repeat this stretch on your other hand.

Static stretch for the anterior deltoid muscles

- Place your hands into the base of your back.
- Drop your shoulders forwards and raise up your chest, as if you're taking in a deep breathe. You should be able to feel a stretch at the front of your shoulders (anterior deltoid).

Static stretch for the deltoid muscles
- Place one arm across the front of your body.
- You can either keep that arm straight or you can bend it to a 90° angle.
- Pull your arm in and towards the opposite arm until you feel a stretch. You should be able to feel a stretch in your shoulder, and slightly in the upper back (rear deltoid, rhomboids and trapezius).

Static stretch for the chest with hands behind the back

- Place your hands into the base of your spine.
- Bring your elbows as close together as possible and push your chest out. You should be able to feel a stretch in your chest (pectoral major, pectoral minor and anterior deltoid).

Static stretch for the chest on a wall
This is a postural stretch for the kyphotic posture.

- Stand beside a wall, with your feet shoulder-width apart.
- Bend your arm to a 90° angle at the elbow, and rest your forearm on to the wall or door frame.
- Place the same-side leg forwards.
- Turn your body and shoulders away from the bent arm until you feel a stretch in your chest (pectoral major, pectoral minor and anterior deltoid).

Static stretch for the lat muscle
- Place your feet shoulder-width apart, and extend one arm across your body in front of you.
- Reach across as far as possible with your hands, while leaning slightly forwards. The key is to try and arch the side of your back.
- You can vary this by holding on to an object or doorway (this will give you a deeper stretch into the lat muscle). You should be able to feel a stretch in the side of your back (latissimus dorsi).

Static stretch for the rhomboid muscles

- Place your hands together in front of you at about shoulder height.
- Reach forwards as far as comfortable with your hands, trying to round the middle/upper part of your back. You should be able to feel a stretch in the middle of your upper back between your shoulder blades (rhomboids).
- It's just like hugging a tree.

Static stretch for the trapezius muscles

This can sometimes help kyphotic postures if you are feeling pain in the neck.

- While looking straight ahead, allow your head (ear) to drop towards the shoulder on the same side.
- Keep your hands behind your back to get the best stretch. You should be able to feel a stretch on the top of your shoulders into your neck (trapezius, levator scapulae).

Ending the myo stretch routine

To finish the routine, stand on your tip-toes and extend your arms overhead nice and straight. You should be able to feel a stretch throughout your body, and then release. Take a little walk around to get the blood moving throughout your whole body, including moving your arms.

You have now completed the myo stretch routine and should feel relaxed, with no tension in your body.